COUNTRIES AND CULTURES OF THE WORLD

IMPERIAL MALADIES

LITERATURES ON HEALTHCARE AND PSYCHOANALYSIS IN INDIA

COUNTRIES AND CULTURES OF THE WORLD

Additional books in this series can be found on Nova's website under the Series tab.

Additional e-books in this series can be found on Nova's website under the e-book tab.

COUNTRIES AND CULTURES OF THE WORLD

IMPERIAL MALADIES

LITERATURES ON HEALTHCARE AND PSYCHOANALYSIS IN INDIA

DEBASHIS BANDYOPADHYAY
AND
PRITHA KUNDU
EDITORS

nova science publishers
New York

Library of Congress Cataloging-in-Publication Data

ISBN: 978-1-53611-863-6

Published by Nova Science Publishers, Inc. † New York

CONTENTS

PREFACE

Literature, medicine and psychoanalysis are now parts of a thriving interdisciplinary field, especially in relation to imperial discourses. Writings by British authors like Rudyard Kipling, Flora Annie Steel, J.G. Farrell, and also by several Indian authors writing in different regional languages can be read in terms of a contested experience in which health and disease, tradition and modernity, politics, gender and psyche come together. Besides, the professional and hermeneutic use of western psychoanalysis in India during the colonial period had its pitfalls especially due to political, cultural and social variations. The revisions that the Indian scholars and practitioners introduced and their subsequent literary representations form a curious and inspiring subject of study which had not hitherto been seriously considered at the academic level beyond the domain of clinical psychiatry. This book engages in an interdisciplinary study of issues like race, medicine, healthcare policies and psychoanalysis in colonial India, with the hope to create a platform for the assembly of and interactive exchanges among such researches in Humanities and Cultural Studies.

The book contains fourteen critical essays, addressing different aspects of imperialism and its interactions with healthcare and psychoanalysis in the Indian context. In his article Debashis Bandyopadhyay has discussed how as a colonial phenomenon the Western notion of psychoanalytic healing evinced potential for reform under the influence of the meditative practices of Buddhism. The time spent by a Freudian psychoanalyst for symptomatic therapy of only sector-specific pathologies could be used economically by Buddhist methods for changing complete personalities as a form of immunity to psychic maladies rather than simply therapies for insidious carcinomas. Freudian techniques show immense potential to adapt to Buddhist forms of restoring peace and happiness in everyday secular life. It is not the absence of sickness that Buddhism aims but aspires to achieve a complete sense of well-being.

Anup Dhar's article examines the concept of Freudian oedipality from an Indian perspective. The notion of the Father both in terms of sexuation and Lacanian Other has been questioned and problematised. Much more fundamental to the study of psychoanalysis is its intellectual basis in Western rationalism that tends to prohibit the child's oedipal cathexes, centred around the triadic relationship with the Father and the Mother. The normative binary of the male and the female in terms of the sexual content of the inter-subjective pattern has been interrogated in a manner that challenges the relevance of Western psychoanalysis in an Indian socio-cultural context. The thesis gains substance from the contributions of Indian psychiatrists like Girindrasekhar Bose and Sudhir Kakar whom Dhar draws on heavily.

Sambuddha Ghosh's article compares the aesthetics of 'malady' in Baudelaire's *Les Fleurs du Mal* and *Paris Spleen* with a Bengali poet and novelist's portrayal of a diseased cityscape of Calcutta in the late 1940s. As a socio-cultural phenomenon 'decadence' is often critically informed by the semantics of a 'disease' which forms the core of diverse, transforming modernities in different human societies. The diverse experiences of a 'flaneur' or ragpicker constitute the 'maladies' of *la modernite* for Baudelaire. The late oeuvre of the Bengali poet Jibanananda Das is likewise replete with metaphors of disease, ailments and overwhelming social anxiety in the face of a decadent Calcutta marked by rampant smuggling, rioting, begging, racketeering, prostitution and the grotesque.The essay seeks to locate the points of convergence and affinities that help us understand how a (post)colonial poet's covert (and overt) use of the metaphor of malady in his late oeuvre captures his impossible longing for a return to a time that was integrative to the human spirit. Jibanananda Das' later works are discussed in relation to the disease of modern life, alienation and existential dilemma which at times lead the readers to a deeper understanding of psychopathological experience.

In her short but insightful article, Chaitali Maitra shows that medicine in colonial India can be understood as a chronicle of the assimilation of Western discursive practices in the otherwise impregnable opacity of Indian cultural scene. Keeping in mind the mercantile concerns, the socio-economic policies and dominance practiced by the existing colonial power, literary masterpieces like *Narsin Hom*, 'Rebati', *Arogya Niketan* and *Putulnacher Itikatha* assumed a significant role in reflecting the social and humanitarian concerns of medicine in the colonial era. Maitra tries to find the fine balance between the difference in attitudes of practising medicine among the villagers, usually living life in a financial crunch. In this particular backdrop, the human approach with a word of kindness goes a long way. However, she also reminds us that the colonial masters used medicine as one of the ways of securing the consent of the masses for its facilities.

Abidita Goswami's article offers a close reading of some short stories by Joseph Rudyard Kipling with a purpose to explore the question of imperial disease concerning different diseases in colonial India and also the various facets of the healthcare remedies taken up by the British government. The chapter focuses on Kipling's attitude towards imperialism as well as towards the diseases suffered by both ends of the colonial system. Goswami also hints at the ailments suffered by Kipling himself, discussing how mental illness has been depicted in his works.

In his article on Amitav Ghosh's *The Calcutta Chromosome*, Pabitra Kumar Rana examines the question of colonial modernity in relation to colonial medicine. He shows how in Ghosh's novel, a critique of colonial modernity takes shape and an alternative, indigenous practice of healing proves to be more successful than the Nobel Prize winning scientist Dr. Ronald Ross' epoch-making discovery of malaria parasite . The novel fictionalises how a group of ordinary native people manipulated Ross towards his discovery. These natives are not merely objects, illiterate and ignorant servants; they are subjects whose object Ross was. Rana argues that this is not Ghosh's reversal of the Subject/Object binary but a dismantling of it. The natives are subjects with a difference: they embark on a navigation of self which is fluid and ever-elusive, and which defies Enlightenment modernity's concept of a holistic and rational self.

Ujjwal Kr. Panda's article presents a comparative study of Graham Greene's *Journey Without Maps* and J.G. Farrell's *The Siege of Krishnapur*. With reference to the recent theories of 'medical humanism', the article shows how the imperial fear of tropical diseases and threatening nutritional conditions that marks the initial days of Greene's journey gradually yields place to a deep-rooted compassion for the patients dying without proper treatment or medicine. Similarly, the outbreak of cholera epidemic in the besieged British garrison of Krishnapur during the 1857 Mutiny in J. G. Farrell's *The Siege of Krishnapur* (1973) is another example of the utter helplessness of the British colonisers faced with the severity of diseases. The two texts, in a way, show the inability of imperial and bio-scientific medical models to cure tropical diseases and, referring to the psychology of the patients, open up the possibility of an intersection of medicine and humanitarian literature.

A curious discourse on Mesmerism in colonial Bengal has been brought to light by Shreya Chakravorty. Her article delves into the 'strange cases' handled by a British doctor, James Esdaile, who used Mesmerism upon the colonial subjects. The doctor's role as an agent of the empire, however, got destabilised when he tried to use the same method upon some European patients and was accused of medical fraud. His contribution to the introduction of this 'anaesthetic' method to alleviate pain during surgeries is undeniable. Yet his implicit faith in the extra-sensory power of Mesmerism sealed the fate of this otherwise promising mode of treatment in colonial Bengal in the first half of the nineteenth century. Esdaile's work on Mesmerism had been a forgotten chapter in the colonial history of psychiatric healing; and Chakraborty's article tries to unearth the reason behind a possibly deliberate erasure of information.

Suvankar Dey's article presents a historical study of tuberculosis in colonial Calcutta. Known as 'Rajarog' or the 'King's Disease' in pre-colonial India, tuberculosis in the colonial period assumes a curious position in the social history of diseases. Supported by documents, writings and reports by the colonial doctors, medical researches and some references made by modern historians, Dey's article claims to be one of the few historical studies that have so far been done in this particular field.

The joint article contributed by Prodosh Bhattacharya and Abhirup Mascharak looks at the portrayal of vampirism, which is a metaphor for homosexuality as disease in Bram Stoker's novel. It then goes on to examine how this view of homosexuality is subverted in a 1949 Bengali adaptation of the novel, only to be reinforced in a subsequent adaptation in 1967. This long and discursive chapter attempts to demonstrate how a medical and psychiatric imagination creeping into the notions of the horrible and dark aspects of human psyche affected the Bengali adaptations of Western horror-stories in colonial and postcolonial times.

Piali Mondal's article examines the use of 'fourth world poison' as a motif in Colonial Bengal's detective stories. Poison can be treated both as stimulant and killer, which has a particular place in the analysis of criminal psychology. Crime fiction claims to have an interesting interrelation with issues of race and empire, and Mondal's paper is a promising addition to the existing scholarship on colonial detective stories.

The fictional and autobiographical works of Flora Annie Steel are taken up by Suchismita Neogi, in order to discuss the psychological outlook of the European women, trying to establish a ground for their behavioural instincts towards the natives. Another aspect that the paper attempts to examine is the connection between imperial anxieties and the tropical health conditions, as experienced from a gendered point of view.

In a joint paper, Sanchayita Paul Chakraborty and Dhritiman Chakraborty attempt to understand the colonial situation in which women as practitioners of medicine had to struggle within the structured and yet subversive spaces based on the intersectional registers of gender and nationalist identity. The authors aptly argue that science in general (and medicinal science in particular) was projected as the major instrument of colonial modernity which entered India with the purported objective of 'civilizing' the mass, thus legitimizing the imperial project. However, the register of women's position vis-à-vis medical and colonial discourses adds a different edge to this whole critique of western science and its trumpeted objective of human development in the colonial discourse, as discussed in this chapter.

The last chapter by Pritha Kundu combines literary and historical approaches. In an attempt to read women's writings and memoirs as 'history', this chapter ventures to follow the journey of two lady doctors in colonial Bengal, namely, Dr. Haimabati Sen and Dr. Jamini Sen, as depicted in their memoirs. The literary genre of 'bildungsroman' thus converges with feminist historiography, and locates the experiences of women medics inside and outside what they understood as 'home'. With reference to some other lady doctors in real life and in fictional representations, the paper also suggests that the boundary between fiction and reality, gets blurred so often.

Finally, the editors of the present volume would like to express their gratitude to all the contributors. Without their co-operation the project would not have been successful. Artless thanks are due to Smt. Chaitali Maitra, Smt. Shreya Chakravorty and Smt. Sanchayita Paul Chakraborty, who not only contributed chapters to the volume, but also helped us in reviewing and editing the manuscript. Things will remain incomplete unless we acknowledge our debt to Mr. Mir Ahammad Ali and Smt. Susmita Haldar, for their generous help in formatting and documenting some of the papers. The Nova Publishers deserve our sincere thanks for taking interest in this academic project. If this book proves to be helpful to our colleagues, fellow-academicians and researchers across the world of interdisciplinary studies, we should consider ourselves fortunate.

January 2017

Debashis Bandyopadhyay
Pritha Kundu

PART 1.
PSYCHOANALYSIS, PSYCHOPATHOLOGY AND THE AESTHETICS OF MALADY

In: Imperial Maladies
Editors: D. Bandyopadhyay et al.
ISBN: 978-1-53611-863-6

Chapter 1

BUDDHA ON FREUD'S DESK: THE EAST SETS FREUD ON A POST-THERAPEUTIC JOURNEY

Debashis Bandyopadhyay*
Department of English, Vidyasagar University, Midnapore, West Bengal, India

Freudian psychoanalysis sought to bring the unconscious mind to consciousness. The process primarily hinged on de-repression and recognition of the fictionality involved in the translation of the Id into Ego. The Ego acts as a false connector between the Id and the Superego. The analyst according to Freud focuses on exploring the act of falsification and intends to bring the patient face to face with reality by entering into his/her unconscious through therapeutic reading of particular symptoms. There is hardly any interest in recovering unconsciousness on a wider expanse beyond the "sector related to the symptom formation" (Fromm 1960, 135). It remains too restrictive to embrace the whole person. The procedural limitations appear to be paradoxical when counted in relation to the

* Corresponding Author's Address: Debashis Bandyopadhyay, 7E Cornfield Road (Ground Floor), Kolkata -700019, West Bengal, India. Email: debashis@mail.vidyasagar.ac.in.

primary objective of Freud: to shift attention to the unconscious mind. Overemphasis laid on instinctual orientation and curing of symptoms stalled the full recovery of the unconscious. Such a recovery is possible if the analyst aims at the total experience of the total man so that the feeling of alienation and the perception of the subject-object split are overcome. This means an immediate grasp of reality without affective contamination and intellection, giving rise to a state of mind where the universal and the social, the unconscious and the conscious merge with a marked attenuation of the affective ego.

A complete de-repression or recovery of the unconscious by consciousness is more radical than the general symptomatic therapy practiced in Western psychoanalysis. The radical aim can be conceived from the perspective of a certain philosophical position, a way of thinking in which absence of sickness is less important than the presence of well-being. Such a sense of well-being can be attained by the consciousness through full and uncontaminated union with the world. This objective is rendered more palpable by D T Suzuki's idea of "the art of living" (Suzuki 1957, 105) and develops from the premises of spiritual humanistic orientation that underlies the tenets of Buddha. Needless to say, the Western Freudian practice was exposed to Buddhist meditative lores during the British rule in India. In fact, a marked exodus of Buddhist concepts to the West began from India and its neighbouring Buddhist countries in the first half of the twentieth century.

Repressive desires grow from a sense of lack and a notion of a split between the self and the other. The Buddhist practice of mindfulness tends to fulfil the lack by a meditative communion with the world uninflected by an attenuated ego. This also includes supersession of the desire to submit to an authority who solves one's problems of existence. The Freudian image of the Father, the idea of paternal prohibition and consequent psychic symptoms like the oedipal complex are consciously overreached in this state of contemplative reality. This is unlike anything that a mother does to a child when it is initiated into the world of the Symbolic language as a normative substitute for its oedipal object of desire. The sense of lack is falsified by words that act as toys and serve as deflective tool for its pathogenic drive. The unconscious passes through a social filter and the reality of the repressed returns through a substitutive metaphor for temporary healing. Jacques Lacan therefore reviewed the alienating world of the Symbolic by defining the Real as a state of the world before it is carved up by language and imprisoned the "barred subject" (Lacan 1977, 52). This does not however mean that language has no therapeutic value; it can when used in an effective way act as a facilitating device for a mindful state of Buddhist *satori*. But the person who only wants to discover the unconscious as a normative cure for sickness will not attempt to achieve the radical aim of complete de-repression or *satori*.

But it would be wrong to suppose that the radical aim has no connection with the therapeutic aim of Western psychoanalysis. In order to cure a symptom and prevent it from recurrence a change of the neurotic traits in the subject is required. And it can be achieved only by pursuing the radical aim of transforming the personality of the subject. The limited aim can be achieved in a limited and less time-consuming method. The elaborate and long-term process that the analyst adopts calls for a more radical aim of complete transformation of the person. It is here that the Buddhist practice renders Freudian psychoanalysis more effective. It is advisable for a person to invest mindfulness in plural identities so that if one fails s/he can still live peacefully by means of dividends reaped from the rest. Plural dispensations in everyday life also help in dissolving any sense of isolation and connecting with the world in its fullness. Freud speaks about this worldly wisdom in unambiguous terms:

> Just as a cautious business-man avoids tying up all his capital in one concern, so, perhaps, worldly wisdom will advise us not to look for the whole of our satisfaction from a single aspiration. Its success is never certain, for that depends on the convergence of many factors, perhaps on none more than on the capacity of the psychical constitution to adapt its function to the environment and then to exploit that environment for a yield of pleasure (Freud 1961, 31)

In spite of Slavoj Zizek's observation of the phenomenon of the disintegrating big Other – "the big Other no longer exists" (Zizek 1991,

12) – in the postmodern world, several political, cultural and economic factors rejig patterns of compartmentalisation in the world and tend to cripple plural possibilities of affiliation by collapsing the expansive world into insular posts of discontent. The Freudian method can address only specific symptoms of such discontent but the Buddhist secular practice of mindfulness can help the subject recreate the implosive plurality in its broadest form and restore the subject's sense of holistic incorporation in the world.

The psychoanalytic method is different from the Buddhist method. It trains consciousness to get hold of the unconscious in a different way. It directs attention to that perception which is distorted; it leads to recognition of the fiction within oneself; it widens the range of human experience by lifting repression. The analytic method is psychological-empirical. It examines the psychic development of a person from childhood on and tries to recover earlier experiences in order to assist the person in experiencing what is now repressed. It proceeds by uncovering illusions within oneself about the world, step by step, so that parataxic distortions and alienated intellectualisations diminish. By becoming less of a stranger to himself, the person who goes through this process becomes less estranged to the world; because he has opened up communication with the universe within himself, he has opened up communication with the universe outside. False consciousness disappears, and with it the polarity consciousness-unconsciousness.

It is important to trace the history of Western enlightenment rationality to discover the suture in an otherwise hegemonic system through which false consciousness entered and contaminated its ideological bearings. Since Descartes split mind and affect and privileged rationality of the mind over the irrationality of physical affect the western subject suffered from a schizoid self. Control of nature by the intellect made man crave for production and acquisition of things. Once Greek and Hebrew wisdom shaped the aim of life as 'perfection of man', the rationality bug now transformed the aim of modern man into 'perfection of things'. 'To have' supplanted the objective of 'to be', while western man, unable to experience affect, became depressed and desperate. In order to allay the anxiety of insecurity stemming from an egotistic exploitation of his environment, the acquisitive man offered lip service to a paternal God who they thought would save them from destruction. The necessity of de-repression of natural affect, felt more intensely when he came in touch with the East, made western man tropicalise affect into institutional ceremonies of monotheistic religions when in reality he continued to pursue the irreligious materialism of his avowed doctrine. False consciousness separated the western subject from his real self.

The Eastern man on the other hand continued to balance affect and intellect in such a manner that they did not suffer the western malaise of isolation so much so that they would feel burdened by the necessity of invoking a transcendent father-saviour in which the monotheistic religions expressed their longings. Buddhism had a rationality and realism superior to that of the Western religions. They could see man realistically and objectively, having nobody but the 'awakened' ones to guide him, and being able to be guided because each man has within himself the capacity to awake and be enlightened, Buddhism helps man to find an answer to the question of his existence, an answer which is essentially the same as that given in the Judaeo-Christian tradition, and yet which does not contradict the rationality, realism and independence which are modern man's precious achievements. "Paradoxically, Eastern religious thought turns out to be more congenial to Western rational thought than does Western religious thought itself" (Fromm 1960, 80).

There was a time when people came to the psychoanalyst to cure their symptoms which often consisted of neurotic obsessions not much different from the one Lady Macbeth suffered when even after repeated washing the blood spots in her hands could not be cleaned. The Doctor of Physic in Shakespeare much before the advent of Freud hardly knew any cure for her disease. Perhaps Shakespeare was a more capable psychoanalyst who expanded the scope of catharsis beyond any specific sector connected with the Lady's symptoms into her total Judaeo-Christian personality contaminated by affective desire. Like Shakespeare's Queen, there were people who wanted to be cured like a sick person would for symptoms like a broken arm, obsession with washing compulsion and various other obsessional thoughts which they could not get rid of. Later people of this sort were outnumbered by 'patients', who functioned socially and did not seem to suffer from any conventional sickness, yet complaining of what came to be known as 'maladie du siecle' caused primarily due to a stultified inner self. These were people whose symptoms were obscure and they would not live peacefully with their selves, complaining of unhappy marriages, insomnia, depression, not enjoying their work and any number of similar troubles. Their obscure symptoms were actually the culturally permissible forms through which they tried to relate their problems, the sources of which actually lay much deeper in their personality. They were alienated from themselves, from their fellowmen and, not the least malodorous, their nature. For these people cure does not consist in the absence of illness but the presence of well-being. The East would contribute generously here; Buddhism has the potential to upgrade Freud's skills to a level Shakespeare demonstrated the need for half a millennium ago.

With regard to the treatment of the individual, Freud was more concerned with a philosophical and ethical aim than he was believed to be. This implicit motivation was consonant with Western rationalism of the nineteenth century which was paradoxically irradiated by "its own interest in and reverence for the irrational, affective side of man" (Fromm 1959, 61). In the Introductory Lectures, Freud speaks of the attempts certain mystical practices make to produce a basic transformation within the personality. He maintains:

> We must admit that the therapeutic efforts of psychoanalysis have chosen a similar point of approach. Its intention is to strengthen the Ego, to make it more independent from the Super-Ego, to enlarge its field of observation, so that it can appropriate new parts of the Id (Freud 1962, 316).

He also sees the role of the analyst in a light which transcends that of the doctor who "cures" the patient. He looks upon the analyst as assuming a superior position than that of his patient and also acting at times as his teacher. The relationship between the analyst and his patient is based not on deception but upon a sincere commitment to truth.

Freud's concept of psychoanalysis transcends the conventional notion of illness and cure. In his idea about the aim of knowledge he echoes the Eastern philosophers. He believes that the power of knowledge is to transform, that theory and practice must not be separated, that in the very act of knowing oneself, one transforms oneself. It is not necessary to emphasise how different this idea is from the concepts of scientific psychology in the last two centuries, where knowledge in itself remained theoretical knowledge, and did not have a transforming function in the knower.

Freud's method has a strong connection with Eastern thought, and especially Buddhism. He did not share the high evaluation of our conscious thought system, so characteristic of modern Western man. On the contrary, he believed that our conscious thought was only a small part of the whole of the psychic process going on in us, and, in fact, an insignificant one in comparison with the tremendous power of those sources in ourselves which are dark and irrational and at the same time unconscious. Freud, in his wish to arrive at insight into the real nature of a person, wanted to break through the conscious thought system, by his method of 'free association'. Despite all criticisms of the content of Freud's unconscious, it has to be admitted that he transcended in an essential point the conventional rationalistic mode of thinking of the Western world, and moved in a direction which had been developed much farther and much more radically in the thought of the East. The other important way in which Freud's devotion to his patients differed from the Western capitalist values of life is the time and care he spent for the treatment of each of his patients. The time he spent for effective healing of a patient's symptom did not by any material standards of value justify the quantifiable character of the effect produced by the treatment. Whereas the qualitative non-Western approach to therapy gains easily from the Buddhist contributions to a sense of well-being in place of specific symptomatic treatment in equal amount of time.

The libidinal drives in human beings are manifested from the time of his birth. The affect so contained in his psychic dynamics is disciplined by reason under the cultural mark of a prohibitor, who in most cases is a father or God. The affective nature under a state of prohibitive repression detaches the man from his true self and contaminates the psyche with inhibited pathogens. One has to understand the difference between inhibition and immunity before any successful management of the instinctual drives is possible. A brief symptomatic analysis of an infant's psychic development from the pre-egoic state to the egoic condition will demonstrate how prohibitive inhibition instead of supporting the immunity power of the consciousness triggers insidious growth of carcinomas in the psychic system and calls for periodical therapies to contain the disease rather than ensure a state of well-being.

An infant in its 'Mirror Stage' (Lacan 1977, 45) identifies with its reflected image in the mirror and yields to the delusion that it is as complete and whole as its mother. But no sooner the infant tries to walk, for example, than it falls down, realizing to its dissatisfaction that it is yet to reach the wholeness of its mother. The sense of pain however is overcome by the presence of the mother holding the infant up and supporting it to walk. With the help of the mother acting like a crutch the infant finally comes closer to championing its futuristic desire for wholeness. This feeling is very complicated in the sense that the infant wishes to be whole and at the same time does not wish so, inasmuch as its falling down ensures the presence of the mother and therefore is a cause for libidinal pleasure to the child. Let us put the idea in an equation: the infant with the help of the mother assumes its wholeness:

Infant (I) + Mother (M) = Whole (W)

Therefore: I = W – M

Therefore: I = Fragment (F), because taking something away from the 'Whole' turns it into a 'Fragment'.

It is clear that the Infant's fragmentariness is both a cause of pain and pleasure. Its desire to unite with the Mother impresses it to prefer the state of fragmentariness, the implications of which are manifested in psychological drives like the desire to annihilate the self and others as a desperate way of escaping from an intolerable sense of isolation and a desire to return to the womb. On the other hand the child also embraces a paradoxical desire to strive for the 'Ideal I' of its imago in the mirror with the help of the developing Ego, which will adjust a part of its Id and place it within an elaborate cultural and linguistic context. The Mother in the equation is now substituted by culturally permissible toys, tropically similar to the reel of wool and the morphemes in Freud's analysis of the 'Fort-Da' (Freud 2003, 52-54) game. A desire for self-preservation or 'eros' is therefore always in conflict with a wish for self-annihilation or 'thanatos'. But both these drives in the developing adult lose their natural character under the prohibitive laws of culture and try to adjust themselves through transference and falsification under the mediation of the ego. In Freud's system of things the prohibitive laws presuppose the presence of a Father who tends to comply with the Judeo-Christian notion of a God. The psychological effect of a superegoic prohibition indirectly buttresses the Ego and creates a symptomatic discontent of obligatory repression in the mind, which would otherwise have functioned more freely in realising the totality of being had the sense of prohibition been absent.

Prohibition stirs a sense of transgression so that compliance to laws becomes less spontaneous. To demonstrate the effect of injunctions on the psyche, Slavoj Zizek turns the cultural paradigm on its head and shows what would have happened to our attitudes had the Laws governing nature enjoined upon us to embrace epicurean dreams instead of puritan disciplines. Zizek cites the example of the effect of injunction on a postmodern subject by referring to the daughter in the comedy *Absolutely Fabulous*. Her mother actively enjoins the daughter to miss school, take drugs, have sex, get drunk, waste money, and so on. This apparently radical behavior, however, terrorises the daughter, leaving her unable to enjoy any of these conventionally transgressive acts. She adopts a thoroughly conservative attitude towards life and 'transgresses' by studying diligently, remaining chaste and sober and by trying to impose a censorious regime upon her mother. For Zizek, therefore, "enjoyment is not an immediate spontaneous state, but is sustained by a superego imperative" (Zizek 1997, 173).

What is common to Jewish-Christian and Buddhist thinking is the awareness that one must give up his will (in the sense of his desire to force, direct, strangle the world outside of him and within him) in order to be completely open, responsive, awake, alive. In Buddhist terminology this is often called 'emptiness', meaning the openness to receive. In Christian terms this is like slaying oneself and accepting the will of God. There seems to be little difference between the Christian experience and the Buddhist experience which lies behind the two different formulations. Instead of making decisions himself, man leaves the decisions to an omniscient, omnipotent father, who watches over him and knows what is good for him. It is clear that in this experience man does not become open and responsive, but obedient and submissive. To follow God's will in the sense of true surrender of egoism is best done if there is no concept of God. Paradoxically, one truly follows God if one forgets about God. Buddhist concept of emptiness implies the true meaning of giving up one's will, yet without the danger of regressing to the idolatrous concept of a helping father. This state of emptiness or 'nirvana' can be achieved through the training of a guide or master, who instead of imposing upon the subject the dictum of perpetually following a superior Law leaves him free to enjoy his satori alone after he achieves the ability to do so. The master disappears after putting things in the subject's own command.

A crucial point of Freudian psychoanalysis is the nature of insight and knowledge which is to affect the transformation of unconsciousness into consciousness. In the first years of his psychoanalytic research, Freud shared the conventional rationalistic belief that knowledge was intellectual, theoretical knowledge. He thought that it was enough to explain to the patient why certain developments had taken place, and to tell him what the analyst discovered in his unconscious. This intellectual knowledge, called 'interpretation', was supposed to affect a change in the patient. But soon Freud had to discover the truth of Spinoza's statement that intellectual knowledge is conducive to change only inasmuch as it is also affective knowledge. It became apparent that intellectual knowledge as such does not produce any change, except perhaps in the sense that by intellectual knowledge of his unconscious strivings a person may be better able to control them – which, however, is the aim of traditional ethics, rather than that of psychoanalysis. As long as the patient remains in the attitude of the detached scientific observer, taking himself as the object of his investigation, he is not in touch with his unconscious, except by thinking about it; he does not experience the wider, deeper reality within himself. Discovering one's unconscious is not an intellectual act, but an affective experience, which can hardly be put into words, if at all.

The importance of this kind of experiential knowledge lies in the fact that it transcends the kind of knowledge and awareness in which the subject-intellect observes himself as an object, and thus that it transcends the Western, rationalistic concept of knowing. Exceptions in the Western tradition, where experiential knowledge is dealt with, are to be found in Spinoza's highest form of knowing, intuition; in Fichte's intellectual intuition; or in Bergson's creative consciousness. All these categories of intuition transcend the split between subject and object. Freud maintained that this split in the relationship between the analyst and the patient dissolves once the former assumes the role of a model or teacher and becomes able to conduct his relationship with the patient which is based on a love of truth. Freud seems to have felt that the analyst has a function transcending that of a physician in his relationship to his patient. But still, he did not change his fundamental concept, that of the analyst being the detached observer – and the patient being his object of observation. In the history of psychoanalysis, this concept of the detached observer was modified from two sides, first by Ferenczi, who in the last years of his life postulated that it was not enough for the analyst to observe and to interpret; that he had to be able to love the patient with the very love which the patient had needed as a child, yet had never experienced. Ferenczi did not have in mind that the analyst should feel erotic love toward his patient, but rather motherly or fatherly love, or putting it more generally, "loving care" (Forest 1954, 23). The analyst understands the patient only inasmuch as he experiences in himself all that the patient experiences; otherwise he will only have intellectual knowledge about the patient. In this "productive relatedness between analyst and patient"(Fromm 1959, 15), in the act of being fully engaged with the patient, in being fully open and responsive to him, lies one of the essential conditions of psychoanalytic understanding and cure.

This humanistic role of the analyst is akin to the role of the master or guide in Buddhist quest for *nirvana* or *satori*, as it is known in its Zen version. The ability to see into the nature of the subject's being, to probe into his unconscious and help him de-repress or move from bondage to freedom, are skills that a Buddhist master would teach a Western psychoanalyst. The Buddhist form of meditation liberates the natural energies in the subject; it prevents him from going crazy or being crippled; and it impels him to express his faculty for happiness and love. Nirvana is not an abnormal state of mind; it is not a trance in which reality disappears. It is not a narcissistic state of mind, as it can be seen in some religious manifestations. According to D T Suzuki, *satori* has a peculiar effect on the person who experiences it:

> All our mental activities will now be working in a different key, which will be more satisfying, more peaceful, more full of joy than anything you ever experienced before, The tone of life will be altered. There is something rejuvenating in the possession of Zen. The spring flower will look prettier, and the mountain stream runs cooler and more transparent (Suzuki 1949, 97-98).

It is quite clear that *satori* is the true fulfilment of the state of well-being which Suzuki described in the passage quoted above. If one tries to explain enlightenment in psychological terms, it is a state in which the person is completely tuned to the reality outside and inside of him, a state in which he is fully aware of it and fully grasps it. He is aware of it – that is, not his brain, nor any other part of his organism, but he, the whole man. He is aware of it; not as of an object over there which he grasps with his thought, but it, the flower, the dog, the man, in its or his full reality. He who awakes is open and responsive to the world, and he can be open and responsive because he has given up holding on to himself as a thing, and thus has become empty and ready to receive. To be enlightened means the full awakening of the total personality to reality. This is not possible under any mark of psychological prohibition or by any means through symptomatic analysis of sector-specific pathologies of repression. The experience of nirvana or satori is not prone to analysis.

References

Forest. Izette de. 1954. *The Leaven of Love*. New York: Harper & Row.

Freud, Sigmund. 1962. "Analysis Terminable and Unterminable". In *Collected Papers V*, 42-61. London: Hogarth.

Freud, Sigmund. 2003. "Beyond the Pleasure Principle". In *Beyond the Pleasure Principle and Other Essays*, translated by John Reddick, 43-102. London: Penguin Books.

Freud, Sigmund. 1961. *Civilization and Its Discontents*. Translated and edited by James Strachey. New York: W.W. Norton & Co. Inc.

Fromm, Erich. 1959. *Sigmund Freud's Mission*. World Perspective series, edited by R N Anshen. New York: Harper & Row.

Fromm, Erich. 1959. "The Limitations and dangers of Psychology". In *Religion and Culture*, edited by W. Leibrecht, 50-81. New York: Harper & Row.

Fromm, Erich. 1960. *Zen Buddhism and Psychoanalysis*. New York: Harper & Row.

Lacan, Jacques. 1977. *Ecrits: A Selection*. Translated and edited by Alan Sheridan. London: Routledge.

Suzuki, D. T. 1949. *Introduction to Zen Buddhism*. London: Rider.

Suzuki, D. T. 1957. *Mysticism, Christian and Buddhist*. World Perspective Series, edited by R.N. Anshen. New York: Harper.

Zizek, Slavoz. 1991. *For They Know Not What They Do: Enjoyment As a Political Factor*. London & New York: Verso.

Zizek, Slavoz. 1997. *The Plague of Fantasies*. London & New York: Verso.

In: Imperial Maladies
Editors: D. Bandyopadhyay et al.
ISBN: 978-1-53611-863-6

Chapter 2

THE OTHER FATHER: OEDIPUS, ANTI-OEDIPUS AND THE AN-OEDIPAL

Anup Dhar*
School of Human Studies, Ambedkar University, Delhi, India

INTRODUCTION

We begin this chapter with what one could call the classical Freudian apparatus and intend to show how the classical Freudian apparatus – marked by the 'Oedipal' – was itself a product of Freud's 'psychobiograph'. Thus, in other words, what appears to be a universal attribute of the human psyche *also* stems from Freud's personal history. In this chapter, I seek to show how 'it' – i.e., Freud's assertion of the universality of Oedipus' fate – stems from, or is an outgrowth, of Freud's "own personal history." Freud writes to Wilhelm Fliess: "I have found love

* Corresponding Author's Address: School of Human Studies (Room No. 60), Ambedkar University, Delhi, Kashmere Gate, Lothian Road, New Delhi 110006. Email: anup@aud.ac.in.

of the mother and jealousy of the father in my own case too, and now believe it to be a general phenomenon of early childhood. … If that is the case the gripping power of *Oedipus Rex* ... becomes intelligible" (Rudnytsky 1987, 7). In that sense, the next section is a kind of psychoanalysis of psychoanalysis.

1. Freud and the Masterplot: The Personal Is (Psycho)Analytical

Sigmund (born 1856) was the eldest child in his family of origin, the first-born son of his rather young mother – Amalie Nathanson – but the third son of his father, Jacob who had previously been married twice with two sons from his first marriage. Therefore Freud had two adult half-brothers when he was born: Emanuel was two years older than Sigmund's mother (who was only 20; Jacob was 40 at the time of marriage in 1855), while Philip was one year younger. Emanuel had one child at the time of Sigmund's birth and therefore Sigmund became an uncle at birth to John, aged one. A niece, Pauline, was born six months after Sigmund. Jacob was thus both father and grandfather at the time of Sigmund's birth. The confusing family picture placed Amalie, Sigmund's mother, in the same generation as his half-brothers. The family atmosphere that contained his parents' trans-generational marriage, the non-diachronic nature of the family series (as if "time is frozen" and each kinship tie has, as if, two names, at times contradictory names; inducing the work of ambivalence) and the "tangling-up of the family sequence" perhaps spawned fantasies/anxieties of plural/conflicting identities for Sigmund, whose genealogical position was very complicated. The situation also fed fanciful fantasies of his half brother being his father. The generations of Oedipus' family line had also become psychically enmeshed when he married his mother and had four children who were also his half-siblings. Freud too was caught up in a generational fault line with his half brothers being of the same generation as his mother. The genealogical confusion is further epitomised by the fact that when his youngest sibling and only surviving brother, Alexander was born in 1866, it was the ten-year old Sigmund who chose the name, thereby arrogating him a paternal function and at the same time unconsciously displacing his father by the half-brother Phillip, since Alexander the Great – after whom he named his brother – was the son of Philip of Macedon (see *Origins* by Jones and Rudnytsky 1987, 16).

2. Freud and the Counter-Thesis/The Other Freud

I also show how Freud himself *exceeds* the standard operating procedure. I show how Freud himself is torn between a 'master-plot'[1] (Brooks 1989 and Jonte-Pace 2001) and a 'counter-thesis' – a counter-thesis different from the *anti*-Oedipal argument in Deleuze and Guattari – a counter-thesis marked by the "maternal corpse in the Freudian corpus" and "death fantasies in relation to the mother, rather than the father, exploring matriphobic and misogynist fears and fantasies, fears of the (uncanny) mother, desires for her death, and fantasies of immortality" (see "Medusa's [*terrifying*] Head" [1922], the *triple goddess* in "The Theme of the Three Caskets", "On Transience" and "The Uncanny" [1919] as also Freud's writings on art, literature and religion; the realms of art, literature and religion often serve as a kind of transferential, if not, *transitional space* [Winnicott, 1972]). The counter-thesis explores anxieties about Jewishness, circumcision, castration and assimilation; it was the *wandering* Jew who was uncanny; lacking home; having perhaps an 'uncanny home' that is simultaneously *womb* and *tomb*; one who is nomadic; and un-homely to the European Christian. It examines our mournful and melancholic encounters with personal loss and social change. It endeavors to *speak the unspeakable* (Jonte-Pace, 2001: 141; Kofman, 1991: 123; Cixous, 1976: 525). The counter-thesis intrudes into Freud's texts in three ways: "some intrusions interrupt and subvert an Oedipal analysis. Others

[1] Masterplot: "it is the fate of all of us, perhaps, to direct our first sexual impulses towards our mother and our first hatred and our first murderous wish against our father. Our dreams convince us that this is so" (see *The Interpretation of Dreams* 1900 SE 4, 262).

explicitly acknowledge the limitations of the Oedipal paradigm. Still others tentatively and hesitatingly begin to develop non-Oedipal analysis" (Jonte-Pace 2001, 3). For example, the plot of *Beyond the Pleasure Principle* differs substantially from the Oedipus masterplot within which the father is interred (Jonte-Pace 2001, 51).

3. Kakar: Counter-Thesis under Erasure

Kakar develops the counter-thesis a little differently; in fact, through this turn to the mother/woman/feminine function (and not just the paternal function) in Indian culture Kakar fractures the counter-thesis itself: "the 'hegemonic narrative' of Hindu culture as far as male development is concerned, is neither that of Freud's Oedipus nor of Christianity's Adam. One of the more dominant narratives of this culture is that of the Devi, the great goddess, especially in her manifold expressions as mother in the inner world of the Hindu son. … Of course, it is not my intention to deny or underestimate the importance of the all powerful mother in Western psychoanalysis. All I seek to suggest is that certain forms of the ["maternal phalanx" or the] maternal-feminine [continuum] [or the "omnipresence of women in the inner world"] may be more central in Indian myths and psyche than in the Western counterpart" (Kakar, 2007, 112); as if, it is not just the household but the inner troubled house of being which is full of women forming in turn an intergenerational caregiver continuum; kind of being-in-the-world-of women.[2] Building on Kakar (who I think puts under erasure the counter-thesis) and Girindrasekhar Bose's works[3], I wish to

[2] Where, however, is the father or the father function then? How is it that the Indian child grows up in a largely maternal-feminine psychological culture and the social culture remains predominantly 'patriarchal'? The psychoanalytic import of the maternal-feminine continuum and the sociological import of the patriarchal, even if fractured, cannot be brought to reconciliation easily or too quickly. Perhaps there is no such thing as an easy relationship between the two. In fact, this shows the tension in the very imagination of the psycho-social; it shows two the hyphen is always an uneasy hyphen.

[3] Here is a representative list of Girindrasekhar Bose's works: (i) Bose, G. (1921). Concept of Repression. Calcutta: Sri Gauranga Press and London: Kegan Paul, Trench, Troubner and Co, (ii) Bose, G. (1931). Gita. In Pravasi. Part 2(1), pp. 9-16, (iii) Bose, G. (1948). A New

develop the fractured counter-thesis in this paper as the 'an-Oedipal' tradition in psychoanalysis; including possible re-readings of *Oedipus Tyrannus* as "the fundamental myth of *knowingness.*" This is important because this conference "is not only about what psychoanalysis can contribute to culture, but about *what culture can contribute to psychoanalysis*" (Lear, 1998, 33). In fact, "if we listen to the culture with an analytic ear, we can gain insight both into the culture and into our fundamental psychoanalytic myths[4]. It is in listening to the culture that [Lear has] found a way to reinterpret the Oedipus myth, the archaic myth of psychoanalysis" (Lear, 1998, 34).

4. Lear: Was Oedipus *Oedipal*?

In his re-interpretation, Lear (1998, 39) suggest: perhaps, we cannot begin to appreciate the meaning of Oedipus "if we continue to think that Oedipus *was* oedipal." One needs to *show* that these events occur *because* Oedipus *indeed has* oedipal wishes. Not only does Freud make no effort to do so—he simply points to the Oedipus myth—there are in the text no hints of oedipal wishes. Of course, as Lear suggests, *if one is already convinced* of the oedipal reading of the Oedipus myth, one will see the entire play as *providing* evidence. However, as soon as one takes one skeptical step backward and asks the question "How do we know that in

---

Theory of Mental Life. Samiksha, Vol 2, No 2, (iv) Bose, G. (1949). Ambivalence. Samiksha, Vol 3, No 2, (v) Bose, G. (1951). The Nature of the Wish. Samiksha, Vol 5, No 4, (vi) Bose, G. (1952). Analysis of Wish. Samiksha, Vol 6, No 1, (vii) Bose, G. (1952). Pleasure in Wish. Samiksha, Vol 6, No 2, (viii) Bose, G. (1952). Sex and Anxiety. Samiksha, Vol 6, No 3, (ix) Bose, G. (1966). The Yoga Sutras. Calcutta: The Indian Psychoanalytic Society, (x) Bose, G. (1980). Svapna. Calcutta: Bangyia Sahitya Parishad, (xi) Bose, G. (1999). The Beginnings of Psychoanalysis in India: Bose-Freud Correspondence. Calcutta: Indian Psychoanalytic Society, and (xii) Bose, G. (2001). Agranthito Girindrasekhar: Girindrasekhar Boser Nirbachito Rachana. ed. Basu, Kolkata: Granthalay Pvt Ltd.

[4] "Myths are isomorphic with the central psychological constellations of the culture and are constantly renewed and validated by the nature of subjective experience." However, given "the availability of the mythological idiom, it is almost as easy to mythologize a psychoanalysis … as to analyze a myth, almost as convenient to elaborate on intra-psychic conflict in a mythological mode as in a case historical narrative mode" (Kakar, 2007: 115).

acting this way Oedipus is acting out *oedipal* phantasies, as opposed to some other phantasy?" one comes to see that the surface evidence of the text points "in another direction." This is because – as Lear shows – Oedipus is not the king. He is *the tyrant.* It is reflected in Sophocles' title *Oedipus Tyrannus,* and it is flattened in the Latin translation *Oedipus Rex,* and then in the English *Oedipus the King.* For Oedipus to be king, he and the Theban citizens would have to understand that he is the son and heir of King Laius. His claim to the throne would then run through his blood. The actual claim he makes on the throne runs through his mind. It is he who solved the riddle of the Sphinx and saved Thebes from disaster. Thebes lacked a king, and they thought there was no heir, so the citizens made Oedipus tyrant by acclamation. For the ancient Greeks, "tyrant" did not only have the negative meaning it has for us today; it also referred to a leader who did not inherit the throne along traditional blood lines. Oedipus gains his position on the basis of his achievements—of *what he does*—rather than on the basis of any given sense of *who he is.* But there is also a sickness in Oedipus' "knowingness": reason is as if being used by Oedipus to jump ahead to a conclusion, as though there is too much anxiety involved in simply asking a question and waiting for the world to answer. The Sphinx had famously asked: "What walks on four legs in the morning, two legs in the afternoon, and three legs in the evening?" But Oedipus walked on three legs in the morning (because his legs were pinned together), limped in the afternoon, and walked on four legs in the evening (blind, he is led by his daughter Antigone). Oedipus is someone who can jump to the conclusion of a riddle and *still* not get it. Oedipus, according to Lear, is suffering from *reflexive breakdown:* he cannot give a coherent account of what he is doing. But he can't focus on the breakdown, and thus remains unconscious of it, because he is too busy thinking. He assumes he *already knows* what the problem is; the only issue is how to avoid it. What he misses completely is the thought that his knowingness lies at the heart of his troubles: what he doesn't know is that he doesn't know (Socrates, on the other hand, was wise enough to know that he *not* a wise man; nobody is; nobody is wise enough). The birth of the tragic is thus not stemming from oedipal desires, but from *abandonment* in infancy and a kind of *compensatory abandon of knowingness*, an abandon of knowingness that renders Oedipus blind to his own unknowingness.

Psychoanalysis from without: Sexuation in Cultural Crucible

The above discussion around (i) Freud's masterplot, (ii) the Other Freud (the counter-thesis), (iii) Kakar's cultural turn and (iv) Lear's somewhat fundamental question (was Oedipus oedipal?) takes us to the doorstep or threshold of two problematics, related albeit. One, given the above, what kind of function would the father come to take, if a culture is not determined/dominated, by what Thomas Lacquer calls the 'two-sex model', where men and women are not seen as the *opposite* sex, but as a *dynamic appositeness* - an unconscious 'see-saw' between gender(ed) identifications; Kakar develops this line of thought – "reading early Indian case histories, one is struck by the fluidity of the patients' cross-sexual and generational identifications. In the Indian patient, the fantasy of taking on the sexual attributes of both the parents seems to have a relatively easier access to awareness. Bose … tells us of a middle-aged lawyer who 'took up an active male sexual role treating both of them as females in his unconscious and sometimes a female attitude, especially towards the father, craving for a child from him. In the male role sometimes he identified himself with his father, and felt a sexual craving for the mother, on the other occasions his unconscious mind built up a composite of both parents towards which male sexual needs were directed; it is in this attitude that he made his father give birth to a child like a woman in his dream … Another young Bengali, whenever he thought of a particular man, felt with a hallucinatory intensity that his penis and testes vanished altogether and were replaced by female genitalia. While defecating he felt he heard the peremptory voice of his guru asking, "Have you given me a child yet?" In many of his dreams, he was a man whereas his father and brothers had become women. During intercourse with his wife he tied a handkerchief over his eyes as it gave him the feeling of being a veiled bride while he fantasized his own penis as that of his father and his wife's vagina as that of his mother " (Kakar, 2007, 111). Let us call this the argument of 'cultural difference', or self-correction of psychoanalytic thinking *from without*. We shall develop this argument in the section on Bose.

Psychoanalysis from within: The Deconstructed 'Father'

Two, what character would this question take if one is considering the question of the father in a post-identitarian frame; when "the Subject is finally in question" (Lacan, 2006, 189). Would we not have to ask '*who/what* is the father'? Lacan problematises the notion of 'father' – Father with a capital F, father as singular in essence does not exist; fatherhood as an all-encompassing idea (a Platonic form) is an illusion (Lacan 1998, 7 footnote). There is thus a multiplicity of fatherhoods, but no essence of "fatherhood" or "fatherliness" (Copjec 2004). Hence we turn to Names of the Father. – Can we re-conceptualise the deconstructed 'father', father under erasure, as nevertheless 'fatherhood without the Father', as 'phallocracy without phalluses', or perhaps, Master's Discourse without the Master? I shall develop the idea of the Master's Discourse without the Master in the section on Lacan; and shall also move from the Master's Discourse to the University Discourse as paradigmatic of the hegemonic father (the father as an upholder of patriarchy). The Hysteric's Discourse – which puts to question the Master's Discourse and the Analyst's Discourse – and focuses on the (object) cause of desire – shall be somewhat more consonant with the father in the maternal-feminine continuum and in situations of the dynamic appositeness of the sexes and of sexuation – *a la* Bose and Kakar.

5. Lacan: Names of the Father

Once one takes the Lacanian Turn, four issues become important:

i. The distinction between the 'always already dead father' and the institution of the Father/Paternal Function is *a posteriori* set on the father's dead corpse; the Symbolic Father is thus also the 'dead father'; the father of the primal horde who has been killed by his own sons; it is, as if, he must be dead so as to be *deified.*

ii. The Borromean Knot of the *Imaginary* (the Imaginary Father is an *imago*, a composite of all the imaginary constructs that the subject builds up in fantasy around the figure of the father ... [which] often bears little relationship to the father as he is in reality); the Imaginary Father can be pictured as an ideal father, the prototype of God-figures in religions, an all powerful protector, or as the terrifying father of the primal horde, *Symbolic* (the Symbolic Father institutes the Law, regulates desire in the Oedipus complex, intervenes in the imaginary dyad between mother and child to introduce a necessary 'symbolic distance' between them. The Symbolic Father is a position in the linguistic and cultural order; it holds more psychological sway than anything flesh-and-blood) and the *Real* Father (the Real Father is of course not the real/actual/living/biological father; it is not the father in a realist sense; in fact, it is the *foreclosed* Father) (see Evans, 1996 and Custodi, 2005; as also Chakrabarti, Dhar and Cullenberg, 2012)

iii. The *Names of the Father* (not Name of the Father). For Lacan, the paternal metaphor marks the beginning of a radically different formative phase in the psychic development of the child. In addition to inaugurating the child's access to the Symbolic dimension by freeing him/her from his/her Imaginary subjection to his/her mother, it gives him/her the status of the desiring subject. The benefit of this acquisition is attained, however, only at the price of a new *alienation*. For as soon as the "speaking being" [*le parlêtre*] becomes a desiring subject, his/her desire is made captive by language and its original nature is lost. From here on it can be represented only by substitute signifiers that transform the object of desire into a *metonymic object*. Thus, for Lacan, the metaphor of the Name-of-the-Father[5] is truly a structural crossroads, with important consequences. Its implications are numerous. When it fails, psychotic processes develop; when it succeeds, it alienates the desire of the subject in the dimension of language by establishing a subjective division (*Spaltung*) that irreversibly separates the subject from a part of itself as the unconscious comes into being.

iv. The reinterpretation of the father in terms of the *Four Discourses*. Who is the father in terms of the Four Discourses? Is the father the 'master of discourse'? What it is to be the 'master of discourse'? Is there a master outside of discourse? Is it possible to establish *sufficient* reason, for a master to be master of discourse, *a priori*? Isn't there always a gap or a leap involved here (which is precisely where the Lacanian hysteric – the *fragile* father, the *nurturant* father, the *feminine* father – subverts and puts to question the master-father) (Lacan's "Four Discourses" in *The Other Side of Psychoanalysis - Seminar XVII*).

This section of the paper tries to make sense of the question of the father in terms of the four discourses. It asks: is the 'function of the father' analogous to the master's discourse and the university discourse (which in short, is the rationalization of the master's discourse; which in other words, is the delusional veil over the master's lack of discourse)? Is the 'function of the father' analogous to the hysteric's discourse (which takes the barred subject as the anchor; which is perhaps subversion through submersion;

[5] 'It is in the name of the father that we must recognise the support of the symbolic function which, from the dawn of history, has identified his person with the figure of the law' (Lacan, 2006: 67). Lacan plays on the homophony of le nom du père (the name of the father) and le 'non' du père (the 'no' of the father), to emphasise the legislative and prohibitive function of the symbolic father. Lacan represents the Oedipus complex as a metaphor in which one signifier (the Name-of-the-Father) substitutes another (the desire of the mother) (see Evans 1996, 122). How this substitution happens in the Indian context, does it happen in this form, is another question?

which puts to question the master's discourse; which shows the limits and the limpness of the master's discourse) and the analyst's discourse (which take the 'cause of desire' as the anchor; and investigates the barred subject's cartographemes of unconscious desire)?

What, however, is Discourse, discourse with a capital 'D' in Lacan ?

> ...what discourse is about, as a necessary structure that goes well beyond speech, which is always more or less occasional. What I prefer, I said, and I even wrote it up on the board one day, is a *discourse without speech*. The fact is that, in truth, discourse can clearly subsist without words. It subsists in certain fundamental relations which would literally not be able to be maintained without language. Through the instrument of language a number of stable relations are established, inside which something that is much larger and goes on much further than actual utterances [*enonciations*] can, of course, be inscribed" (Lacan 2007, 13).

Lacan (2007 [1969-1970]) unlike Foucault talks of only Four Discourses. Lacan's focus is on structure rather than content; Lacan asserts: "There are structures – we cannot describe them in any other way" and there is a "fundamental relation", "the one I define as the relation of one signifier to another. And from this there results the emergence of what we call the subject" – the paternal subject – "via the signifier, which ... functions as representing this subject with respect to another signifier" (Lacan, 2007, 13). When speaking, the content would be what is said whereas the structure could be understood as the relation between the agent who speaks and the other they address. Indeed, agent and other are two of four positions central to the theory of the Four Discourses. These positions always occur in the same order (see Figure 1); the *truth* motivating the *agent* to address the *other*, which results in a *product*.

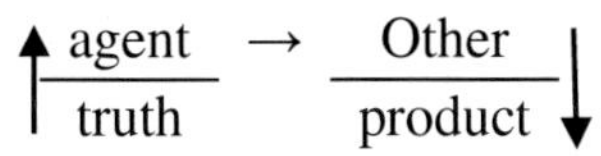

Figure 1. Four-footed apparatus.

These positions provide the matrix or fundamental structure of Discourse. How an agent relates to, or addresses, another person can differ and would presumably depend on that agent's motivation. As such, there are a number of terms that can occupy these four positions (see Figure 2). For Lacan, the master signifier, knowledge, divided subject, and *objet petit a*, are the only four positions and, as if the positions occur in a loop, the terms are always in the same order. That is, if the master signifier is first, in the position of *truth*, then knowledge will be second, in the position of *agent*, with the divided subject in the position of *other* and the term *objet petit a* in the position of *product* (University Discourse; see Figure 2) but if the master signifier is last, in the position of *product*, then knowledge will be first, in the position of *truth*, etc. (Analyst's Discourse; see Figure 2). As the order of the terms does not change for Lacan, there are only four possible ways in which the terms can be arranged in the four positions, which gives us the Four Discourses; The Discourse of the University, The Master's Discourse, Hysteric's Discourse, and the Analyst's Discourse.

Four terms:
master signifier (S_1)
Knowledge (S_2)
objet petit a (a)
divided subject ($\not{S}$)

University Discourse

$$\frac{S_2}{S_1} \rightarrow \frac{a}{\not{S}}$$

Master's Discourse

$$\frac{S_1}{\not{S}} \rightarrow \frac{S_2}{a}$$

Hysteric's Discourse

$$\frac{\not{S}}{a} \rightarrow \frac{S_1}{S_2}$$

Analyst's Discourse

$$\frac{a}{S_2} \rightarrow \frac{\not{S}}{S_1}$$

Figure 2. Four Discourses.

The Discourse of the Master can be seen in terms of *authoritarianism* where a dictator (master signifier) issues orders. While someone who is subject to these orders (barred subject) may know what they need to do they will not know why. That is, they will not know what (truth) motivates the dictator and in obeying the dictator's commands they will never really know what they are producing (*objet petit a*). In the Discourse of the Hysteric, the cause of the hysteric's symptom (the *objet petit a*) is unconscious, the hysteric is a barred subject who addresses the Other (the master signifier) in order to understand their symptom (truth), and the knowing they bring about (truth) is not related to what caused their symptom (*objet petit a*). The Discourse of the University is common to education where the master signifier is unconscious original knowledge that supports the knowledge that is to be taught, and the knowledge that is to be taught (truth) addresses the student (*objet petit a*) as lacking knowledge (barred subject). In the Discourse of the Analyst, the analyst's knowledge (truth) leads them (*objet petit a*) to address the patient (barred subject), which elicits knowing (master signifier) from the patient that is not connected to the knowledge in the analyst. What then is the 'father'? Which Discourse is the father's discourse?

What then is the *function* of the father in the Indian context? *Who* is he? Or more pertinently *what* is he? Does a dialogue between Lacan (Four Discourses) and the works of Bose and Kakar help us make sense of the father in the Indian context? Is he just a concrete-real entity with a life history? He is, of course. Is he an Imaginary entity? He is, perhaps, as an internalized Other. Is he a Symbolic entity, an entity marked by the Name(s)-of-the-Father; an entity that embodies law-morality-rules-taboo functions and the 'categorical imperative', an entity whose rule is rendered more profound in his absence, in death; the Indian widow comes to be circumscribed by the law of the patronymic much more after the death of the father-to-her-child? Why? How does this happen? Why is the Symbolic father – the father recalled in an everyday sense our morning prayers in missionary schools – "*in the name of the Father, holy be your Name*" – much more menacing than the father in the concrete-real? What are the cultural antecedents of this Symbolic father? What is the genealogy of the father-function in our 'inner worlds'? How does the Indian child relate to the father? How do we make sense of the ambivalent scream of the Indian child: "Father, can't you see I am burning (with desire)"? As if, the Indian child is torn between a foregrounding of "I am burning" (I have in mind female foeticide) and "I am burning with desire"; as if the father is to take note of both the pain and the desire; both the fact that "a child (in us) is being beaten" and the fact that "a child (in us) is deviating from the beaten track of desire."

Further, what is the role of the *pita*, the *pitri-purush* in our lives? Figure of authority, figure of the taboo function, figure of the spectral, the spirit, the *bhuta/preta* after death, the Indian child continue to be haunted by the multiple functions of the father, perhaps the ten heads/apparitions of the father. Further still, what is the difference between the father-function marked by *Moses and Monotheism* – where the son renunciates desire-gone-awry by ritual circumcision – and the father-function marked by *pitamaha* Bhisma who himself is the (sexual) renunciate par excellence? The father in the Indian mythic tradition is repeatedly seen to be cursed by blindness, by sexual impotence, by the curb on sex; and all these emerge as a complex configuration of functions of vulenerability; and yet the Indian father at times becomes the embodiment of the 'holy war' against the Muslim Other. How then do we make sense of *paternality* in the Indian context? How do we understand the 'father' in his many apparitions? How is the father-function related to the mother-feminine-woman continuum in the Indian context? Could the Indian father be seen as embodying a dynamic movement between the four positions in the Four Discourses?

6. THE INDIANS: MINOR LANGUAGE?

> … psychoanalysts today seems to stand out more particularly in terms of their divergences, resulting from different conceptions about the mind, but also because of the differences stemming from their cultural traditions. Lacan's work could only have evolved in France, and I believe that Winnicot's work is intimately related to what he owes to his native land. (Green 1986, 4)

The section takes off from Derrida's (somewhat uncharacteristic[6]) assertion in *Geopsychoanalysis: "... and the rest of the world"*: "there is practically no psychoanalysis *in* Asia, or in the South Seas" (Derrida 1998, 69). One would like to ask: is it because 'psychoanalysis has never set foot' on Asian soil? Or is it because *here* psychoanalysis "has never taken off its European shoes"? Is it because as Derrida says "African [or Asian] psychoanalysis was European, structurally defined in the profoundest way by the colonial state apparatus"? Is it because much of Asian or African psychoanalysis were "merely emanations of what we used (how accurately!) to call "metropolitan" organizations" " (1998, 69). Derrida however could have put to examination this somewhat *unguarded* statement. One could have put to examination the nature of the shoe, the nature of the foot, the shoe-foot relation. One could have found out whether the foot did manage to walk barefoot, even if, for a while, or whether the foot did manage to fashion some 'Other' footwear, other than the European 'One'. Between barefoot walking and walking with exclusively European footwear there are a number of intermediate possibilities, in-between possibilities that are not exactly midpoints.

It is in this context that Spivak's three questions (*Psychoanalysis [out] in Left Field and Fieldworking*) become important: one, "given radical iterability, how have the right-handed hitters in India dealt with the pitcher they perceived to be the scientific dominant discourse of psychoanalysis"? Two, "can *we* perform conventions laid down according to Hebraic and Hellenic stories"? Did we? Three, is the parricide story the "beginning of human history"? Does not Freud foreclose possibilities of looking at a *different* (rather than *deviant*) language game by relegating "matriarchal polytheisms" to the "pre-history of humankind" or by making Islam an "abbreviated repetition of the Jewish religion"?

[6] Derrida says: "I don't know whether you will find such considerations trivial or shocking" (1998, 69).

Spivak as if hands over the question of what happens "out in the left field" to Asish Nandy. What do we make of Nandy's legitimate lament in "Towards an Alternative Politics of Psychology": "what changes over time are the microtheories, not the *architectonics* of western psychology"! (2004, 335) Nandy shows how the problem is thus not just of universalism; the problem is deeper; and *non-critical cultural relativism* is not the antidote to universalism. Cultural relativism "makes of the various Asias and Africas a colourful cluster of "national origins" where a rhetorical version of psychoanalysis - with its "anthropological origin", and "religious origin", and its story of subject-construction - can find a field (Spivak in Shamdasani and Munchow 1994, 45). Non-critical cultural relativism, which constitutes the ethical core of conventional cross-cultural psychology or, for that matter, humanistic psychology is thus not the antidote.

> Such relativism was originally a response to the indiscriminate universalism that mirrored the parochial cultures in which the social sciences had grown. And it was supposed to correct the bias of the first generation of social scientists, often drawn from among Christian missionaries and colonial bureaucrats. But political processes are made of more resilient stuff than conceptual innovations in the social sciences. And the idea of cultural relativism was soon co-opted by that particularism which the relativism was supposed to fight. Even in their more sophisticated versions, most cross-cultural and humanistic psychologies see modern psychology as a transcultural reservoir of knowledge and other psychologies as its handicapped cohorts waiting to be interpreted by and integrated with the world of modern psychology. The other psychologies thus become, definitionally, mixed bags of good and bad insights and good and bad data. The good in them are to be swallowed by modern psychology, the bad rejected. Neither cross-cultural nor humanistic psychology, despite the best of intentions, can grant alternative psychologies the right to integrate within the latter what they see as the best of modern psychology and to reject the bad.
>
> The implication of seeing the non-modern psychologies as sacks of isolated insights or data is that these insights and data can then be used to ornament, strengthen or alter the micro-theories of modern psychology.

> The basic paradigms and culture of modern psychology remain untouched and are, in fact, carefully adapted to new empirical facts. What changes over time are the microtheories, not the architectonics of modern psychology. (Nandy 2004, 335)

This paper therefore asks: what happens when psychoanalysis and 'India' come close? What happens to psychoanalysis when it is (played) *out in the left field*? Far off from the metropolis? Does India become the *analysand* and provide to western psychoanalysis 'case material' about the aboriginal world? Or does India change the architectonics of western psychoanalysis? What was the nature of ab-Original psychoanalysis? Was it psychoanalysis turned upside down? Or was it the other side of psychoanalysis?

Was it inaugurating, as Bose would suggest, "a *new* theory of mental life" and of 'sexuation', a theory *different* from the one offered by psychoanalysis in the original, a theory marked by insights drawn from what gets reflected in the 'rearview mirror', namely insights from the Yoga Sutra and the Bhagvad Gita, a theory "open still to intervention and the carving out of a practice that is responsible by volleying responses rather than imposing an alien science"(Bose 1994). Or was it *Indian* psychoanalysis? But in which sense was it 'Indian'? Was it the 'Indian logic' of the psyche? Or was it the logic of the 'Indian psyche'? Taking off from an extant logic of the Indian psyche (exemplified by epic manuscripts like the Mahabharata as against Greek Tragedy) was it offering to the west the Indian logic of the psyche (and not just the logic of the *Indian psyche*)?

The options are therefore these:

1) Retain the Universal
2) Displace the Universal – make an Indian version out of the Universal – the Universal Indian. We thus have an Indian version of psychoanalysis – 'Indian Psychoanalysis' – we have an Indian version of the Oedipus Complex – our bodies, our psyches, our

myths are different – we have the *Ganesha Complex* – here the son does not kill the Father – here the Father (Shiva) kills/castrates the son (Ganesha). However, through this displacement, Oedipus Complex is retained as the fundamental logic of the psyche.

3) Have many displaced versions of the Universal – U1, U2, U3, U4 …
4) One can look at this displacement in two ways: (a) one can rejoice in this displacement – one can see this as *post*-colonial. (b) One can also see this as the hidden power of the western universal – that it is retained as universal even in its displacement or through its displacement – such that 'our modernities' are in the last instance 'modernities' – modernities nevertheless.
5) What if castration complex is not the constitutive node/anchor of human psychic life? Does the text of the human psyche take a peculiar turn when one takes the Bhagvad Gita (as against the 'Sophoclean theatre') as the manuscript of human culture, as Bose had done? What if one builds on the transcript of the Kurukshetra? What is the configuration of the psychic that gets scripted in the Mahabharata? Can it usher in and inaugurate the thinking of another psychology – a psychology different from what the west could think of – given its obsession with Greek tragedy?
6) What if Bose's psycho-logic was radically different from Freudian psychoanalysis?
7) What if Bose was not a *savage* Freud?
8) One can then provincialise the Universal – such that the presumed/purported Universal is only a contingent particular (P1). There are a number of particulars – Freud is one particular (P1) – Bose is another (P2). In the Bose-Freud correspondence, these particulars come face to face for dialogue; as if P1 is in dialogue with P2.

Bose-Freud Correspondence

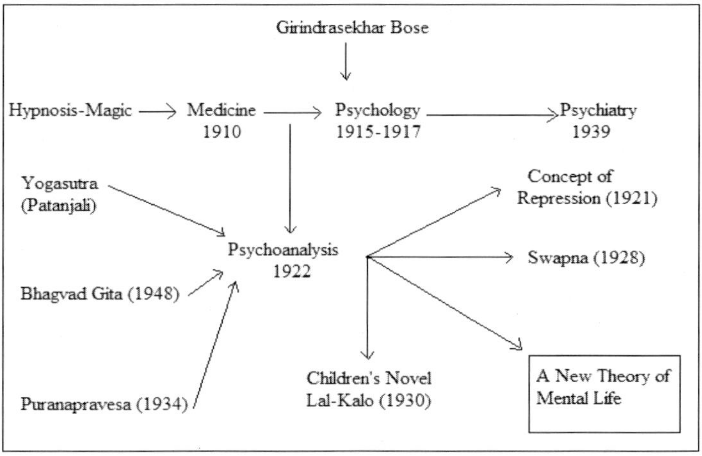

Figure 3. Bose-Freud Correspondence.

Girindrasekhar had established communication with Freud: "I take the liberty to send you under separate cover a book entitled *The Concept of Repression*" (*Bose-Freud Correspondence*, 1999, 1). Freud had also acknowledged receipt of the book: "I acknowledge the receipt of your book … and am glad to testify the correctness of its *principle views* and the good sense appearing in it. … It is interesting that *theoretical reasoning and deduction does play so great a part in your demonstration of the matter, which with us is treated rather empirically*" (1999, 2). Freud in a letter dated 20th February 1922, further added:

> It was a great and pleasant surprise that the first book on a psychoanalytic subject which came to us from that part of the world (India) should display so good a knowledge of psychoanalysis, so deep an insight into its difficulties and so much of deep-going original thought [as if such insight was not expected of the nat(i)ve!]. Dr. Bose has singled out the concept of repression for his inquiry and in treating this theoretical matter has provided us with precious *suggestions* and intense motives for further study. Dr. Bose is *aiming at a philosophical evolution and elaboration of our crude, practical concepts* and I can wish,

> psychoanalysis should soon reach up to the level, to which he strives to raise it. (Freud 1999, 7)

Once again, the west is *crude practical* and the east *philosophical.* Is this humility? Or is this a condescending pat on the back? We come to know from a letter dated 31st January, 1929 that Girindrasekhar had sent once again some of his own works to Freud:

> I would draw your particular attention to my work on Oedipus Wish where I have ventured to *differ* from you in some respects. … I also enclose a Bengali book on dreams, which I have just published. … Please accept the book as a token of my deepest regards for the *Father of Psycho-analysis.* (Bose and Freud 1999, 14)

How would Freud respond to the dent in the theory of the Oedipus that Bose was trying to institute? Here Bose is trying to re-think the particularities of the "[Sexed] Subject who is finally in question" (Lacan 2006, 229) in psychoanalysis. However, he is not just trying to move out of the particularities of the sexed subject of analysis in its Judeo-Christian moorings. He is also hinting at a different understanding of Oedipality (and not just at a relativist version of psychoanalysis), an understanding marked by what he called, the *shifting* Oedipal Point (1950, 72). The Oedipal Point was for him a possible moment in the evolution of the sexed subject. However, this moment is preceded by 'mother identification' and 'passive homosexuality' in at least the boy child (Bose also argues that the Oedipus Point in the girl child develops earlier than in the boy and the identification with the mother is more intense. The original form of homosexuality is active in the female and passive in the male). For Bose, the homosexual disposition is one of the earliest to appear in the course of analysis. In its order of emergence it either precedes the Oedipus or immediately follows it. Further, for Bose the "desire to be a woman is the primitive form on which the castration idea depends" (1950, 74) and castration idea is what keeps the Oedipus in check (1950, 75). Thus there is a *double dialectic*: on the one hand, between the homosexual disposition (within which there is a dialectic between active and passive) and the Oedipus Point and on the other, between the Oedipus Point and the Castration Idea (within which there is a dialectic between the 'wish to be woman' and the 'wish to be man'). But how would Freud respond to this critique and obeisance, critique masked in obeisance? Freud in a letter dated 9th March 1929 acknowledged the receipt of Girindrasekhar's works:

> You directed my attention on the Oedipus wish … *In fact I am not convinced by your arguments.* Your theory of the opposite wish appears to me to stress rather a formal element than a dynamic factor. I still think, you underrate the efficiency of the castration fear … I never denied the connection of the castration wish with the wish to be a female nor that of the fear with the horror of becoming a female. … But I confess I am by no means more convinced of the validity of my own assumptions. We have not yet seen through this intricate Oedipus matter. We need more observations. (Bose and Freud 1999, 16)

Girindrasekhar wrote back on 11th April 1929:

> Of course I do not expect that you would accept off-hand my reading of the Oedipus situation. I do not deny the importance of the castration threat in European cases; my argument is that the threat owes its efficiency to its connection wish the *wish to be female*. The real struggle lies between the desire to be a male and its opposite the desire to be a female. … The Oedipus mother is very often a combined parental image and … I have reasons to believe that much of the motivation of the 'maternal deity' is traceable to this source. … My theory of the opposite wish is not a mere formal philosophical statement as you suppose it to be. … it gives the exact dynamics of repression when a particular wish is pushed into the unconscious; it explains the mechanisms of imitation, retaliation, conscience, projection, etc. … The theory of the opposite wish will explain the occurrence in pairs in the same individual of such traits as sadism and masochism, observationism and exhibitionism etc. … (Bose and Freud 1999, 17)

With respect to the Oedipal Point, Bose asks whether homosexuality is a primary psychological trait and which form – the active or the passive, is the more primitive one. For Bose, in the case of the male child the mother, on whom a part of the libido has already been fixed, is looked upon as a person of the same sex. The Oedipus love becomes thus tinged with homosexuality and there is an 'irradiation of identification'. The interests of the mother now become the child's interest by the mechanism of irradiation; the child looks upon the objects of his mother's interest from the standpoint of the mother. This results in the expansion of the child's ego and ultimately leads to the appreciation of the characteristics of his new objects of interest. His identification goes with a passive, sexual attitude towards the father. This is the first phase of homosexual development in the boy and precedes the true Oedipus point which comes later. The passive sexual attitude towards the father is thus originally a true feminine attitude. The appreciation of the father's characteristics means an unconscious identification with the father and the father has a two-fold relation, one with the mother and the other with the boy himself. These attitudes are the counterparts (opposites) of the previous attitude towards his father viz. (i) in the situation of identification with the mother and (ii) independent of such identification respectively. The former is responsible for the first hetero-sexual love which is directed towards the mother; and the latter for the homosexual love of the active type which is directed against the father in the first place and acts also as a defence against the original passive attitude. Elements of 'gross sexuality' are thus to be observed in the feminine attitude of the boy towards the father and also in the subsequent active attitude towards the mother. In point of time so far as gross sexuality is concerned in the boy under ordinary conditions of family life, the passive homo-sexuality, which is here another name for the feminine attitude is the first to develop and is directed towards the father. Next in order of development are the active homosexual attitude towards the father and the heterosexual trend towards the mother. These two are more or less coexistent. The true Oedipus Point therefore comes after the identity with the father has been established. The true Oedipus Point is characterized not only by love for the mother but also by hatred towards the father. The genesis of hatred is to be sought for in the homosexual attitude of the boy towards the father.

Under normal conditions of family life, the psycho-sexual development of the girl proceeds in a slightly different manner. The first identity with the mother leads, as in the case of the boy, the development of a passive sexual attitude towards the father. The first sexual love therefore, is heterosexual and is of passivity. As this is directed against the father the Oedipus Point develops earlier than in the case of the boy. Later on when the identification with the father has been established, the girl begins to love the mother in an active homosexual way. The first homosexual love of the girl is therefore of the active type and in order of development dates later than the first passive homosexuality of the boy. The other aspect, corresponding to the active homosexual phase in the boy, leads to the appreciation of the active hetero-sexual male trait. The development of passive homosexuality in the girl can only come as a defense against the active homosexuality directed against the mother just as the homosexuality in the boy is a defense against the primitive passive homosexuality directed towards the father. The defense is traceable to the functioning of the opposite wish by identification.

Freud wrote back on 12th May 1929 …

> I am fully impressed by the difference in castration reaction between Indian and European patients and promise to keep my attention fixed on the problem of the opposite wish which you accentuate. … I wonder what the relation of the opposite wish to the phenomena of ambivalence "may be" … (Bose and Freud 1999, 19)

Here is Freud's relativism – "I am fully impressed by the difference in castration reaction between Indian and European patients"(19); Indian and European patients are different; they have different reactions; psychoanalysis would need a slight tweaking in Indian conditions; it would be *tropical psychoanalysis*; grant the devil her due; grant Bose cultural relativism; but hold on to the universal. Here is Freud's attempt at holding on to psychoanalysis as a transcultural reservoir of knowledge. In this structure Bose's psychology becomes, definitionally, a mixed bag of good and bad insights and good and bad data; the good are to be swallowed, the bad rejected. But Freud, despite the best of intentions, cannot grant Bose the right to integrate within aboriginal psychology what he sees as the best of psychoanalysis and reject the bad. In the process, the basic paradigms and culture of modern western psychoanalysis remain untouched and are, in fact, carefully adapted to new empirical facts. What changes over time are the micro theories, not the architectonics of modern Western psychoanalysis.

In addition, is Girindrasekhar Bose rendering redundant the importance of the phallus that has been paradigmatic of much of psychoanalysis? In other words, Bose moves from having or not-having an (part) object to be*ing* or not-be*ing* (like a) subject; he is moving from *possession* (and hence the consequent pride, envy, anxiety) to identification with a momentous Other; he is moving from the notion of a cannibalistic or devouring self to an image of self where the self extends itself outwards towards Others through identification, where Others are mirrors and not objects. It is not just an argument for cultural relativism. It is not that Indian and European patients are different in psychic disposition. It is that the phallus is not the fundamental object or signifier of sexed subjectivity. India is not an analysand who offers different case experiences to phallocentric psychoanalysis. India is an analyst of the European obsession with the phallus (and the Oedipal) as the structuring principle of psychic constitution.

Freud writes back again on 1st January 1933:

> … the theory of the opposite wishes strikes me as something less dynamical than morphological which could not have been evolved from the study of our pathological material. *It appears to me flat so to say, it seems to lack a third dimension.* I don't think it is able to explain anxiety or the phenomenon of repression. … we did neglect the fact of the existence of opposite wishes from the three sources of bisexuality (male and female), ambivalence (love-hate) and the opposition of active-passive. These phenomenon have to be worked into our system to make us see what modifications or corrections are necessary and how far we can acquiesce to your ideas. (Bose and Freud 1999, 24)

Girindrasekhar explains further his differences with Freud with respect to (1) the unconscious or complex wish (*avadamita iccha* or *gudhaisa*), (2) the resistance (*badha* or *pratibandha*) and (3) the censor (*prahari*). For Girindrasekhar this censor is the opposite wish of the repressed one:

> According to Freud … shame, hatred and fear represses our wish and unconscious feelings like Love, Violence, Jealousy can influence us without our knowledge … but I think in the unconscious, only wishes exist; … this wish has a dynamic character in our mind. … In fact, shame and fear is the result of particular repressed wishes, they are not the cause of repression. … an opposite wish to our sexual wishes holds us back from being sexually attracted towards our relatives. … if the resistance is only external, then our wishes wouldn't have remained unconscious. Because external resistance cannot drive a wish from the conscious. To do that, we need another wish. So the main reason for not having a sexual wish towards our relatives, is having an opposite wish … (Bose 1966)

Bose takes his argument forward in the re-interpretation of the *Bhagvad Gita*:

> All traditional sacred texts have as their main objective, the desire to resolve [internal] grief [*atyantik dukkha*]. Desire for *moksa* (ultimate liberation) is also driven by a wish to resolve grief or pain … The ideology and means of resolving grief is quite different in the Orient and Occident. The West teaches: make yourself capable of struggling in society; while competing with others … change your surroundings according to your convenience. In this thorn ridden society, try to uproot as many of them as you can. ... the *sanatan* (age-old/traditional) ideology here teaches us something else: you will never be able to uproot all the thorns, so you must build yourself in a way that you are not hurt by the thorns. It is better to wear a pair of shoes instead of attempting to sweep away all the stones and dust from the road. One ideology tries to overcome nature; the other tries to overcome and discipline the Self … (1948)

The works of Girindrasekhar Bose (1886-1953), the first sa*va*ge psychoanalyst, has thus served as an example of critical acceptance of (a) received theory of the mind in colonial India. Bose re-read psychoanalysis as another version of "the older theories of consciousness in India" and thus transformed the "introspective project of Indian philosophy into a new prose of liminal psychoanalysis" (Nandy 1995). "(T)he tenets which Bose formulated, despite having Freudian traits, were notably different. … The world of dreams is made available for another explanation by a non-western psychoanalyst, whose interpretation makes the 'wish' a dialectical and dynamic category" (Basu 1999). What was then the contour and nature of our 'critical engagement' with received theories of the mind (here Freudian psychoanalysis)? What was the nature of our reception of western theories? What was the nature of our critique of psychoanalysis? Was Bose's 'new theory of mental life' focused on the 'constitutive ambivalence of (gender) identification' (as opposed to attachment) the ground, the *Grundrisse* for an external critique? While for Freud, the ground of sexed subjectivity and sexual development is one of attraction, for Bose the ground is one of *identification* and the *irradiation of identification.* Also, while for Freud the change from sadism to say masochism is a change in the object (and not a change in the aim), for Bose these are changes in *aims/wishes* and not just changes in objects. Is Bose's 'New Theory of Mental Life' then the opposite wish of its European counterpart? And then does the concept of unity proposed by him provide a compromise between this opposition? Does Bose (and Kakar) emerge as the dynamic an-Oedipal *third* (a third Freud thought was absent in Bose's work) between Oedipus and anti-Oedipus?

In search of the *cause*, Bose looks at an *internal compass* marked by the see-saw of the double wish and the *dwaita-ta* ('two-ness', like the Irigarayan 'two lips'; and not *dwitva*, or binarisms) of ambivalence-internalization, where each marks difference with respect to the other. Bose's new theory is marked by an expressed dynamic – the *see-saw of opposed wishes.* It is marked by an interiority of ambivalence or an ambivalent interiority. It is also marked by a belief that a harsh super-ego or social taboo cannot be the *only* cause of repression. There must be something in the psyche to accrue to such a moral injunction. In that sense, Bose proposes a particular/new theory of the mind. Does Bose, in the process, institute a radical semantic change, or perhaps a scandalous anti-semantics that is supposed to have marked the coming of psychoanalytic language? Does Bose give the figure of a wish shadow, that which follows, follows the Other, sticks tenaciously? Are *two* of the wishes, in perpetual embrace, in deconstructive catharsis? What is psychoanalysis? What is the psyche? Repository of *ghost effects* or *crypt effects*? Is it a *hauntology* (as against ontology)? Is it about the *sexual spectral* that follows son, follows father?

Thus the double wish and the see-saw form an unending circuit of ambivalent identification, which in turn creates another double: the double of ambivalence and identification as constitutive of the human subject and the unity principle (as against the pleasure principle); where the Lingam itself is a gender ambivalent Form; as if difference is kept alive even in identity. In Bose's framework, the Father is not the castrating authority. Castration doesn't come from without. It comes from within. The castration wish is inside. It is in the desire to be female.

In the West, identification is about Identity. In Bose, identification is about Unity. In Bose, identification does not lead to I becoming You, but I and You becoming One. This One or the principle of Unity is the third in Bose. Through Opposite Wishes Bose develops a theory of cancelling out; and then he moves to a higher synthesis through the principle of unity. The Bose-ian analyst plays the role, becomes the embodiment of the 'repressed Opposite Wish' in the patient's psyche.

7. Oedipus, Anti-Oedipus and the An-Oedipal

Indeed, *Oedipus Rex* is perhaps *the* preeminent classical text in the Western tradition. For, more than two millennia before *The Interpretation of Dreams*, Aristotle in the *Poetics* identified *Oedipus the King* as the bench mark for excellence in tragedy. Evidently, Aristotle's grounds for admiring *Oedipus* were in many respects from Freud's, though in point of

> fact the convergence between their views is deep and startling: Aristotle's emphasis on the plot accords with Freud's remarks on the way the play's action "can be likened to the work of a psycho-analysis"; Aristotle's key concepts of *anagnorisis* ("recognition") and *peripeteia* ("reversal") suggest the aims and method of psychoanalytic therapy; and Aristotle shares with Freud the conviction that the most painful tragedies are those where the family members are involved. But overriding these specific areas of agreement is the simple fact that Aristotle joins with Freud in adopting an *Oedipus-centered* perspective, and hence in elevating Sophocles' tragedy to its unique place in the life of the Western mind.
> (Rudnytsky 1987, 337-338)

When one takes *Oedipus Rex* as the text of the psychic and not just as a text of the social/historical (however radically one may read it – as Jonathan Lear does so well) we would end up with a narrative of 'acts committed in the context of non-knowledge/ignorance' (Oedipus did not know who his parents were), remorse/guilt at what one has done, self-chastisement or sacrifice to atone for one's deeds (Oedipus blinds himself). This core/originary 'guilt-ridden traumata' sets/marks off the 'psychic teleology'. Freud tries to make a case for such a psychic teleology in Moses and Monotheism.

However, if one takes the Bhagvad Gita as the text of the psychic one gets a different psychic teleology – a psychic teleology sparked off by an affront to a menstruating woman in the blind king's court of justice now being avenged by the collective of husbands she has; however there is a catch or halt or deferral to this seamless narrative; one of the five husbands is haunted by a near-primal doubt that could be so characteristic of the conception of dharma (what should I do?) and why not the human (who am I?) as well; the doubt is premised on the question: can I kill? Not ordinary killing. Can I kill my relatives, my brothers, my teacher, my grandfather even if I am here to avenge the trauma inflicted on 'my' woman? The answer was "yes, you have to" to forestall further harm and auxiliary destruction by a group of marauding men.

While the premise is guilt (what have I done? The 'should' and 'should not' being known beforehand) in the Oedipal narrative, the premise is dharma (what should I do? Should I kill? The 'should' and 'should not' needs reflection) in the narrative of the Bhagvad Gita; even the call of dharma (the a-dharma woman has been subjected to) requires further reflections on dharma (avenge an originary a-dharma done to women); it is, as if, dharma sparking off further reflections on dharma. While in the Oedipal narrative the psychic teleology is sparked off by 'guilt' *a posteriori* (guilt after the event), in the Bhagvad Gita the psychic teleology is sparked off by 'reflection' on self and dharma *a priori*.

The choice is thus not between Oedipus (a la Freud) *and* anti-Oedipus[7] (a la Deleuze-Foucault).

---

[7] (i) Deleuzo-Guattarian philosophy accuses psychoanalysis of not allowing for a conception of subject-hood beyond the Oedipal triangle. (ii) It believes this imperialist signifying function is intimately connected to our capitalist structure, which necessitated Oedipus as structuring meta-narrative in order to assure that we lack, that our desires cannot be fulfilled. Their fight against capitalism produced a methodology with which to question its truth, which can equally be applied to psychoanalytic reasoning. (iii) To Deleuze/Guattari, the fixing of drives is the consequence of the formation of a fixed order of society. The repressive structure of society preserves a fixed order of drives by excluding certain desires. Whereas Freud defines drives as being repressed by reality, as in the Oedipus complex. For Deleuze/Guattari, this reality is social repression in itself. There is, for example, no primal instinct towards incest. for Deleuze/Guattari, this lack is constructed by society. Society's mode of repression is structured by Oedipus, effecting, thereby, the coincidence of social and psychic repression. (iv) Unlike psychoanalysis, which regards the body as a developmental union or aggregate of partial objects, organs, drives, orifices, each with their own significance, their own modalities of pleasure which, through the processes of Oedipal reorganization, bring these partial objects and erotogenic bodily zones into alignment in the service of a higher goal than their immediate, local gratification (the ultimate goal being reproduction), the Bodies without Organs (BwO) invokes a conception of the body that is disinvested of fantasy, images, projections, representations, a body without a physical or secret interior, without internal cohesion and latent significance. BwO does not refer to a body that is literally without organs, but a body that is not determined by its organs, not structured or ruled by them as in psychoanalysis, where predetermined instincts, genitals, sensualities are the basis for Freud's theories of sexualities and drives. (v) How is Oedipus inscribed into our subjectivities? In a despotic society it is through incest itself that the despot's power is justified; the despot's power is based on a myth that escapes coding. Through this overcoding of incest as the origin of society, the despot stands outside of the tribal socius. Marrying queen and mother, he creates a mythical alliance with mother earth, and therefore makes himself into the father of the tribe. Incest is beyond the taboo: it becomes the origin of that which necessitates the incest taboo in order to keep existing. (vi) The modern version of the despot is capitalism: money has become the new omnipotent almighty. (vii) If there is a triangle mother-father-Oedipus, that was created by psychoanalytic reasoning, the same is applicable for capital-labour-resources. Capitalism breeds the capitalist worker, like money creates money, like language creates irrational and rational sounds, or, in our case, gender binarism creates male, female and hermaphrodites. Deleuze/Guattari argue that although the family remains outside of economic production in capitalism, as capitalism is not dependent on the social form of the family anymore,

The choice is not just between "pre-oedipal in the child, exo-oedipal in the psychotic, para-oedipal in others" (Deleuze and Guattari 2000, 51)

The task perhaps is to look for non-Oedipal or an-Oedipal psychic economies (a la Bose and Kakar).

Does this then offer interesting insights for 'another' or even a 'new theory' of mental life; a minor language *from* (and not just *of*) India? A minor language relevant to both east and the west; this new language/theory could be represented as having been born in the east or as having been borne by scholars residing in the east and texts belonging to the eastern shores.

References

Basu, Amit. 1999. "The Coming of Psychoanalysis in Colonial India: The Bengali Writings of Dr. Girindrasekhar Bose." *Occasional Works.* Calcutta: Centre for Studies in Social Sciences.

Bose, Girindrasekhar. 1921. *Concept of Repression*. Calcutta: Sri Gauranga Press and London: Kegan Paul, Trench, Troubner and Co.

Bose, Girindrasekhar. 1931. "Gita." *Pravasi.* Part 2(1), 9-16.

Bose, Girindrasekhar. 1948. "A New Theory of Mental Life." *Samiksha* 2. 2: 108-205.

Bose, Girindrasekhar. 1949. "Ambivalence." *Samiksha* 3.2: 54-75.

Bose, Girindrasekhar. 1951. "The Nature of the Wish." *Samiksha* 5.4: 203-214.

Bose, Girindrasekhar. 1952. "Analysis of Wish." *Samiksha* 6.1. 1-11.

Bose, Girindrasekhar. 1952. "Pleasure in Wish." *Samiksha* 6.2: 53-69.

Bose, Girindrasekhar. 1952. "Sex and Anxiety." *Samiksha* 6. 3: 191-200.

Bose, Girindrasekhar. 1966. *The Yoga Sutras.* Calcutta: The Indian Psychoanalytic Society.

capitalism is dependent on the family as a psychic formation. Its structure is mere simulation: the father stands for capital, the mother for resources and the child for labour force. The naturalness of capitalism is hence re-emphasised by the naturalness of gender binarism. Bose and Kakar both problematize gender binarisms.

Bose, Girindrasekhar. 1980. *Svapna*. Calcutta: Bangyia Sahitya Parishad.

Bose, Girindrasekhar, and Sigmund Freud. 1999. *The Beginnings of Psychoanalysis in India: Bose-Freud Correspondence.* Calcutta: Indian Psychoanalytic Society.

Chakrabarti, A., Dhar, A. and S. Cullenberg. 2012. *World of the Third and Global Capitalism.* New Delhi: World View Press.

Deleuze, Gilles, and Felix Guattari. 2004. *Anti-Oedipus: Capitalism and Schizophrenia*. London: Continuum.

Derrida, J. 1998. 'Geopsychoanalysis: and "the rest of the world"', in C. Lane (ed.) *The Psychoanalysis of Race.* New York: Columbia University Press.

Freud, Sigmund. 1957. "Moses and Monotheism." *The Standard Edition of the Complete Psychological Works of Sigmund Freud.* Trans. & ed. James Strachey. London: Hogarth.

Irigaray, Luce. 1985b. *This Sex Which is Not One*. Ithaca: Cornell University Press.

Kakar, Sudhir, and Katharina Kakar. 2007. *The Indians: Portrait of a People*. New Delhi: Penguin-Viking.

Kakar, Sudhir, and John Munder Ross. 2011. *Tales of Love, Sex and Danger.* New Delhi: Oxford University Press.

Kakar, Sudhir. 1982. *Shamans, Mystics and Doctors. A Psychological Inquiry into India and its Healing Traditions*. New Delhi: Oxford University Press.

Kakar, Sudhir. 1989. *Intimate Relations: Exploring Indian Sexuality. New Delhi:* Penguin India.

Kakar, Sudhir. 2011. *A Book of Memory: Confessions and Reflections*. New Delhi: Viking Penguin.

Lacan, J. 2006. *Ecrits.* Translated by Bruce Fink. New York, London: W. W. Norton and Company.

Lacan, J. 1977/1998. *The Four Fundamental Concepts of Psychoanalysis*. New York: W. W. Norton and Co.

Lacan, J. 1998. *The Seminar of Jacques Lacan.* Edited by Jacques–Alain Miller. *Book XX. On Feminine Sexuality: The Limits of Love and*

Knowledge ... Encore (1972-1973). Translated with notes by Bruce Fink. New York: W. W. Norton and Co.

Laquer, Thomas.1990. *Making Sex: Body and Gender from Greeks to Freud.* Cambridge, Massachusetts: Harvard University Press.

Lear, Jonathan.1998. *Open Minded: Working Out the Logic of the Soul.* Harvard University Press.

Nandy, Ashis. 1995. *The savage Freud and other essays on possible and retrievable selves.* Delhi: Oxford University Press.

Nandy, Ashis. 2004. "Towards an Alternative Politics of Psychology." In *Bonfire of Creeds: the Essential Ashis Nandy.* 324-328. Delhi, India: Oxford University Press.

Sinha, Tarun 1954. "A Short Life Sketch of Girindrasekhar Bose." *Samiksha*, Bose Special No., edited by Nagendranath Dey. 62-74.

Spivak, Gayatri. 1994. "Psychoanalysis in the left field and fieldworking: Examples to fit the title." In S. Shamdasani, & M. Munchow (ed.), *Speculations after Freud: Psychoanalysis, Philosophy and Culture.* London: Routledge.

In: Imperial Maladies
Editors: D. Bandyopadhyay et al.
ISBN: 978-1-53611-863-6

Chapter 3

'DEEPER MALADIES ON HARRISON ROAD': THE AESTHETICS OF ILLNESS IN BAUDELAIRE AND JIBANANANDA DAS' LATE OEUVRE

Sambuddha Ghosh*
Department of English, Krishnagar Government College,
Krishnagar, Nadia, West Bengal, India

"This life is a hospital where each patient is possessed by the desire to change his bed."

Charles Baudelaire, *Paris Spleen*

INTRODUCTION

The persistent conflict between the aesthetics of the 'here-and-now'—fluid, ephemeral and ever changing—and a larger sense of 'historicity' is a persistent feature among the otherwise different 'modernities' we have

* Corresponding author's address: Krishnanagar Govt. College, College St., Krishnanagar, West Bengal 741101. Email: sambuddha.puspendu@gmail.com.

inherited from Europe. As subjects altered forever by the certainty of colonial contact, we are members of a populace that has seen their inherent subjectivity being aptly fragmented and refracted through the lens of diverse, contesting modernities that found simultaneous co-existence in our shared histories of nationalism, political 'independence,' partition, post-war alienation, and finally, a succinct (but arbitrarily constructed) semantics of 'disease' and 'decadence.' In Baudelaire's Paris, the possible trajectories of exploring the annals of mid 19th century urban space provided him with alternative 'ways of seeing' through which, as Foucault tells us, it was possible to understand modernity as "a break with tradition, a feeling of novelty, of vertigo in the face of the passing moment" (Foucault 1984, 43-44). However, Foucault hastens to add that it is not just any attitude embodied in the flux of such widespread socio-cutural displacement, it is a form of rebuttal directed towards the temporary, "the will to "heroize" the present" (Foucault 1984, 45). But this is also an ironic disposition towards the present.

For indeed, the rhetorical tropes of keen observation, so apparent in Baudelaire's conception of the several iconic figures of modern life were distinctly differentiable in their respective particularities. Benjamin and Foucault have both observed—albeit in different contextual paradigms—the intellectual process by means of which Baudelaire understands modernity primarily as a set of paradoxes which need to be reconciled by assuming varying stances in the face of incessant change: that of the *flâneur*, the *dandy* and the *artist*.

It is the object of this paper to read these ideological predilections with reference to the late oeuvre of the 20th century Bengali poet Jibanananda Das. I wish to demonstrate how an identifiably unique nexus of comparison exists between these two very different poets otherwise removed in time and geographical space in the broader context of two contesting, and mutually dependent 'modernities' they inhabited. I am certainly not the first to identify this nexus. Dr. Sanjay Mukhopadhyay's Bengali article 'Harrison Road ey aro Gobheer Awshukh' ('Deeper Maladies on Harrison Road') (Mukhopadhyay 2011) tacitly explores how these two subjectivities, themselves fragmented by their disparate legacies of geography, class and time can be thought of as converging upon each other. Dr. Mukhopadhyay's article shall become my point-of-departure from whence, I can perhaps take a new flight and try to answer a few questions about the extent to which an 'aesthetics of malady and illness' collectively informs their discourse. The methodology I have tried to adopt is that of comparing aspects of Baudelaire's and Jibanananda's work in the retrospective light cast on them by arguments outlined by Georg Simmel in 'The Metropolis and Mental Life.' Simmel illustrates how the Parisian cityscape during the First Empire produced a distinct 'neurosis' in perception. In the face of a rapidly transformed cityscape which presented the constant paradox of coexistence—that of imposed bourgeois 'order against the violently suppressed 1848 Revolution—the individual's right to his own unique identity was put at stake by a post-industrial society bereft of older social values (Simmel 1903 (2000), 1999-2005). Likewise, politico-economic changes constitute the real foundations upon which the tumultuous decade of the 1940s affects Jibanananda's city, Calcutta. I will try to direct attention to four major 'spaces' which make up this strange epistemic and rhetorical overlap between the two poets: the shared familiarity of (a similar) economic and historical context, a shared, and comparable form of 'gazing' that delineates the namelessness of locale, the notion of *time as historicity* and finally, the metaphor of 'illness and malady' that results from a peculiarly 'modern' experience of the metropolis.

The late oeuvre of Jibanananda Das deserves close textual reading in order to locate these shared social, political and cultural moorings. For this very purpose, I shall analyse, following Dr. Bhattacharya, poems such as 'Beggar,' 'Night' or 'Shores of Existence' where the poet had, probably for the first time in his poetics, come to terms with the metaphor of urban modernity as a 'malady' in his poems through well-developed conceits ('Night'), indicative asides ('Beggar') and witty dialogue ('Lighter Moments'). The iconic crystallisation of his alienated aesthetic expositions seems to have happened in the year 1948, where in the space of four months, Jibanananda finished writing three full-length novels: *Jalpaihati* (April-May 1948), *Sutirtha* (May-June 1948) and *Malyabaan* (June 1948).

All of the three novels are marked by the traces of man's encounter with the maladies of *la modernite* displaced to a hybrid and partly cosmopolitan colonial city marked by American troops, Swedish doctors and Marwari businessmen. It will then go on to answer a larger question that Derrida raises in the context of cultural (re)appropriations: Is it possible, given the differences in 'historicity' in two contexts so far removed in time, to identify a criterion of historical 'iterability,' one which "both puts down roots in the unity of a context and immediately opens up this non-saturable context onto a recontextualisation' (Derrida 2003, 26).

I. The Ironic Disposition: *La Modernite* and the Metropolis

The 'quality' of the stance assumed towards the immediacy of the ephemeral 'present' can be understood to determine to what extent the observer in *Paris Spleen* or *Les Fleurs du Mal* situates and suits himself to either of these roles:

a. At one end of the prism Baudelaire locates the "*flâneur*," the man of modernity who has ample time on his hands, goes on strolling through city-streets and builds up a moving storehouse of memories. Solitary and gifted with an active imagination, he is afloat with the general tide of effervescence that characterises the present.
b. Pitted against the *flâneur*, Foucault identifies the solitary figure of Constantin Guys, the 'Painter of Modern Life' *par excellence*, whose disposition towards the 'contemporary' is that of ironic detachment. In other words, for Baudelaire, Guys embodies that familiar paradox, where European modernity's consistent attempts to come face-to-face with its own estimation of the present finds its body-double, a radical scepticism with regard to the principle of the 'contemporaneous.' While the 'quotidian' is valuable for its

own sake, Foucault finds in Baudelaire's unveiling of the Parisian cityscape a will "to imagine it (*la modernite*) otherwise than it is, and to transform it not by destroying it but by grasping it in what it is" (Foucault 1984, 44). This is revealed in the stance taken by the *dandy* in the face of social and economic change.

c. This ironic attitude embodied in the general philosophy of *dandysme* was read by Foucault as a deliberate one. Through the dandy's refusal to accept the present "as it is," he initiates a process of self-elaboration that is at once 'ascetic,' 'free' and one which plays on the transfigurations of a peculiar ethical attitude. These do not "have any place in society itself, or in the body politic. They can only be produced in another, a different place, which Baudelaire calls art" (Foucault 1984, 45)

If contradiction (between the 'interminable present' and nature of *dandysme*) is the first principle which aligns Baudelaire's schema of envisaging *la modernite* to the sense of a split subjectivity, the second is the presence of melancholia as a defining characteristic of personality. Herein lies the dandy's paradoxical 'originality' - "the affliction [of] melancholia arising from an ineffable feeling of having been wronged" (Hadlock 2001 - 2002, 58). The dandy was someone who never took part in any social labour, and (unlike the *Bohemians*) they were not just content to enjoy a carefree, indolent lifestyle where one simply rejected bourgeois values. This was because, despite their attempts to "cultivate the same chance existence, the same love of inactivity, the same appetite for celebrity," they were different in that "one was handsome and given to elegance, the other prided himself on being ugly and affected a careless exterior" (Seigel 1986, 104). But *dandysme* consisted in more than this. "The dandy is, in effect, a mournful figure, but one mourning some locus of signification that has been *cathected* onto his body, but is forever unknown to him" (Hadlock 2001-2002, 59), and upon this riddling co-existence of opposites stands the self-fashioning of the dandy. This is also apparent in the dandy's overt insistence on artifice, "a compelling need to transcend nature" (Seigel 1986, 104) and his retreat into a symbolic domain. The emphasis on deliberate gallantry not only connoted freedom to him, it had a bearing on his outward appearance of irreverent aristocracy which had "bearing, pretension, and disdain" for the dull and the commonplace (Seigel 1986, 99). Artifice was important here, as a necessary means to transcend the realities imposed by Nature. The figure of Constantin Guys who spent years as a reporter and a war correspondent for the *Illustrated London News* during the Crimean War becomes revelatory to Baudelaire for these very reasons. Like the dandy, he "has a horror of blasé people…" and records the effervescent instantaneity of the present moment like a 'man of the crowd,' unnoticed. (Baudelaire 1965 (1863), 5-6). *Paris Spleen* is therefore poised between the 'prosaic' nature of modern life and the 'poetry' born out of a philosophy of neglect that nonchalantly stands in opposition to it:

> By 'modernity' I mean the ephemeral, the fugitive, the contingent, the half of art whose other half is the eternal and immutable…This transitory, fugitive element, whose metamorphoses are so rapid, must on no account be despised or dispensed with. By neglecting it, you cannot fail to tumble into the abyss of an abstract and indeterminate beauty, like that of the time the first woman before the fall of man. (Baudelaire 1965, 13)

The Hausmann Renovation of the Parisian metropolis added new boulevards, cafes, streets and museums to the city's earlier design. However, Baudelaire's artistic sensibility drew him contrapuntally, "irresistibly towards the city's bright lights, beautiful women, fashion, luxury, its play of dazzling surfaces and radiant scenes while his Marxist conscience wrenches him insistently away from these temptations, instructs him that these whole glittering world is decadent, hollow, vicious, spiritually empty, oppressive to whole proletariat, condemned by history" (Bermann 1982).

The old debates pertaining to the question of what 'modern' might denote ('contemporaneous,' 'of a similar time' or even better, 'that which is always contemporary, so that, in essence it becomes eternal') are important to consider here. It is this strand of thought that will allow us to examine 'thematic,' as well as 'formal' similarities in diction between the two poets.

For Jibanananda, the experience of comparing the time he spent in his native Barishal to his wanderings within the labyrinths of Calcutta becomes deeply invested with an 'ambivalent' meaning. The 'forties' in Calcutta were a tumultuous decade, ravaged by the horrors of the Second World War and the pangs of Partition which effectively 'dispersed' large populations across national borders. Towards the beginning of the decade, there was a general feeling of 'resentment' in the political climate of Bengal about the legitimacy of 'constituional' (the Congress) over 'violent' (the undivided Communist Party of India, or a few 'other' nationalists) means in the nationalist struggle. The war years in Bengal saw an infamous famine in 1943, a direct consequence of the Japanese invasion of Burma and the increased demands for food made by the British Indian Army stationed at Bengal. Despite a better than average crop in 1943, food shortage was rampant. Churchill's refusal to ship supplies to India meant that the famine was 'man-made.' His action was to be seen in the context of his wanting to send aid to civilians of Nazi-occupied Greece who were also going through a famine (Herman 2009, 513). He noted that the "starvation of anyhow underfed Bengalis (was) less serious than that of sturdy Greeks" (Wheatcroft 2014). The *petit-bourgeois* class comprising of 'middle' tradesmen manipulated market conditions to earn an overwhelming share of 'speculative profits.' The spectre(s) of smuggling, racketeering, pimping and the threat of Hindu-Muslim riots loomed large over a city that had suddenly acquired a 'cosmopolitan' character. The poet's native Barishal could never match up to the sheer variety of experiences that would meet him in the course of his endless 'strolling' along the city's dark underside. He was without a full-time job during the latter part of the decade and worked as a life insurance agent during the period. The memory of his older, and more sublime Barishal was already a thing past. His experience of charting the moribund lanes and alleys of colonial Calcutta is thus evocative of an alternative *flânerie*. In the Bilingual webzine *Parabaas*, Dr. Sanjay Mukhopadhyay draws attention to the most enduring and popular photograph of Jibanananda, one in which his eyes are directed 'elsewhere,' looking outwards from the frame, fixed on something distant, 'over there.' The penetrative and searching stare is more than the right of the individual poet to be lonely, it is in tune with Baudelaire's conceptualisation of the observer as 'a prince enjoying his incognito wherever he goes' (Baudelaire 1965 (1863), 14). In a striking passage Mukhopadhyay notes:

> In his earlier years, Jibanananda wrote in a poem called 'Lonely Autograph': "Oh you know not—and yet/All my songs are directed to you." There appears to be a clever punning on his part when he uses the Bengali word 'lokkho' which means both 'directed to' and 'observe.' What appears to be an offering of romantic love changes forever if we consider the second connotation of the word. To 'observe' is to be on camouflage, which is also a treacherous form of gazing. This rather ponderous mask of anonymity allows him to extract a heightened sensitivity towards the sights and sounds of the metropolis. Whatever constitutes what (one) has written has been recorded by someone else, someone other than me. This implicit inclusion of the 'observer consciousness' in me within the world of my observations is a legacy of 'historicity'—immediate, ephemeral and therefore, 'modern.' (Mukhopadhyay 2011, my translation)

II. "Beneath the Sky, Like a Vast Canopy…": The Namelessness of Locale

If the corresponding socio-historical contexts inhabited by the two poets are indeed comparable, so is their 'gazing.' For Jibanananda, permanently exiled to a turbulent Calcutta in 1946 and not technically a "refugee," finding suitable housing and jobs proved to be a difficult task. "[H]e got none of the concessions extended to refugees," and struggled constantly for the last seven years of his life trying to find a teaching job. (Seely 2006). He had arrived in Calcutta to try his hand at journalism and the move had proven to be a disaster. He was appointed the editor for the

Sunday section of Bengali daily, *Swaraj* in 1947, and was sacked within the same year.

Jibanananda's vision of the streets and narrow lanes of the metropolis is informed by a certain implacable dissociation from the category of the 'particular.' When for example, in the poem 'City' he writes of the "(h)earts of countless travellers/Forever search in desperation, their way not found," Jibanananda is not speaking of just Calcutta, even though it is the material constraints of the particular city that are acting on him. More than the 'geographic' nature of the locale, he is abstracting the experience of the metropolis, Calcutta is a labyrinth born out of his intellect. This echoes Baudelaire's lines in 'The Ragpicker's Wine' where "(t)he jumbled vomit of enormous Paris" makes the drunkard ragpicker dither between the two mutually overlapping worlds of the 'Spleen' and the 'Ideal':

> He takes great oaths and dictates sublime laws,
> Casts down the wicked, aids the victims' cause;
> Beneath the sky, like a vast canopy,
> He is drunken of his splendid qualities.
> (Baudelaire 1982 (1857), 113)

As I have already noted earlier, *Mahaprithibi* (1945) appears to be the fulcrum against which Jibanananda's late verse turn decidedly cryptic and somewhat intelligible. The narrative voice is scrupulously observant of sights and sounds, and often has a searching intent, just as the narrative voice in *Paris Spleen* maps the city as 'imagined,' watching the silent procession of faces that "...do not resent the ferocious beast hanging around [their] and glued to [their] backs" ('Crowds'/Baudelaire, 1970 (1869)). Jibanananda's 'Night' is a poem in a similar textual vain, this is precisely that point in his oeuvre when he discovers that 'other' city through its medley of sound-image scapes:

> Lepers open the hydrant and lap some water.
> Or may be that hydrant was already broken.
> Now at midnight they descend upon the city in droves.
> Scattering, sloshing petrol. Though ever careful,

Someone seems to have taken a serious spill in the water.
Three rickshaws trot off, fading into the last gaslight.
(Das, 'Night' (1948) trans. Clinton B. Seely)

This is followed by a promise to 'defiantly' turn away from 'Phear Lane,' for miles stopping only '[o]n Bentick Street, at Teritti Bazaar' where the night air appears to him 'dry, as roasted peanuts. The unique signature of his angst-ridden language here seals off successive conceits, confronting the reader with disparate, tableaux-like scenes of a Jewish girl rapt in song, a throng of 'Firangi youth' walking past, and an 'old Negro smiling/Cleaning his briar pipe with the still faith of an old gorilla' (Das, 'Night'). Such episodes of night life had found their way into Jibanananda's poetry as early as the decade of the 1920s, but the late poems are marked by a resolute will to reach that 'elsewhere' in the life of the metropolis; they are laden with a precise *historical consciousness* in a way that former poems are not. Just as in *Paris Spleen* (originally published in 1869) where Baudelaire's poet-persona is ever willing to explore the poorer neighbourhoods of Paris, Jibanananda uncovers 'the incomparable privilege of being able to be himself or someone else, as he chooses' (Baudelaire 1965, 15). The relatively 'poor' and 'questionable neighbourhoods of Rajabazaar, Chitpur, Phear Lane and Burrabazar are brought out in the newly evolved diction of the Bengali Modernist whose exposure to the Occidental 'exotic' was verily qualified in his ability to synthesise his reading habits to the world of lived human experience that was, in turn, surrounded by a heightened historical awareness. One needs only to compare epithets and syntanctical word-combinations in Jibanananda's late verse to observe how he freely switches his register of speech, making the unlikely verbosity of jarring village dialects stand together with sophisticated conceits. Let us compare two poems, Baudelaire's 'The Eyes of the Poor' with Jibanananda's 'Beggar' to understand this better. Baudelaire's poet-narrator situates the weary 'old fathers' reflections on beauty and contrasts them to those of his son in the poem 'Eyes of the Poor':

> The eyes of the father were saying: "How beautiful it is! how beautiful it is! one might say that all the gold of our poor world is painted on these walls." - The eyes of the little boy: "How beautiful it is! how beautiful it is! but this is a house that only grants entry to people who are not like us." (Baudelaire, 'The Eyes of the Poor,' 1869, 52)

Lyrical incomprehension motivates the disjuncture between the thoughts of the poet' and his 'beloved.' Sitting at a 'new café on a new boulevard,' the woman chides the mindless perspicuity of the poet, citing how the poor look 'insufferable with their eyes open like carriage gates.' This is at jarring odds with the narrator's own version of things, where "(he) felt shame at (their) glasses and carafes" which, he thinks, are bigger than their thirst. In 'Let's Whack the Poor,' he hurls himself at a beggar who accosts him on the streets, kicks him, knocks him in the eye and urges the beggar to fight back because the only way one can establish a relative equality with the beggar is through the exchange of equal violence, which is preferred to the humiliating servitude of being a 'supplicant.' The beggar retaliates and 'beats [him] to a pulp,' knocking off four of his teeth, after which the narrator salutes him as his 'equal' and offers him 'the honour of sharing (his) purse' (Baudelaire 1869, 97).

If we now consider Jibanananda's 'Beggar,' we shall notice how the narratorial voice seems to follow the movements of a beggar through the nefarious multitudes of the city, and does not fail to observe his unsettling loquacity:

> One pice I got from Mathkotha,
> And another from Pathuriaghata,
> If I can get just one more,
> My rice comes husked from the paddy-mill."
> With this—his face, protruding—the gaslight beams,
> Among the crowd, the deeper maladies on Harrison Road—
> A world's wrong, from a beggar's blunder; a world full of flaws.
> (Das, 'Beggar,' 1942, my translation)

III. THE "ENDLESS DARK OF SUNLIGHT": MALADIES OF TIME AND HISTORICITY

What could be read as a 'spiritual malaise' of 'a civilisation' in its 'wrong' but man's encounter with 'decadence' at a historical era replete with 'bourgeois' values? Yet, as I will try to show in the next section, the metaphor of 'malady' in Jibanananda's late oeuvre is not just conceptual. At the level of plot construction, this metaphor is mercilessly externalised through the gripping paranoia of strange and 'inconceivable' diseases and the spectre of an old, decrepit body-politic ailed by the 'dark malaise' of a historical inheritance that was doubt-ridden and perverse. In his 'surreal' poems such as 'Horse,' the perverted causality of the "weird dynamo of this Earth" appears not to disturb the "primordial craving for grass" in Moheen's horses who are in essence, presumed to be no different from "neolithic horses in the moonlight' (Das, 'Horse,' 1948, self-translated). The individual man's personal access to Time and History is exhausted at the moment of his death, but the quality of the 'lived experience' of Man across generations may be surmised and judged—or at best evaluated—, through a series of 'historical touchstones,' and only in a retrospective light.

It is useful to look into Jibanananda's notion of 'time *as* historicity' as illustrated by Faizul Latif Chowdhury. He makes an interesting point when he tries to examine the extent to which the array of temporal references in Jibanananda's diction are denotative/specific over the puny mass of 'generic' connotations in his poetic oeuvre that delineate a general sense of 'historicity'[1]. These select few (generic) temporal references are the ones

[1] "That in Jibanananda reference to specific time or period often carries no direct documentary or attributive meaning can be further discussed with regard to 'One Day Eight Years Ago'—one of the most celebrated poems of Jibanananda. The poet narrates the story of an unexplained suicide that apparently took place eight years ago. That the suicide took place eight years ago is mentioned nowhere except in the title of the poem. Notably it is 'eight' years—not 'nine,' nor 'seven.' Why eight? A curious reader may inquire if there is any clue to a personal episode hidden in the temporal reference of the title. It is important to observe that nothing of the text—no word or meaning—would change at all if the poem's title was altered to 'One Day Five Years Ago,' replacing 'eight' with 'five.' However, the title as it is, or even with the change in time reference, connotes a recollection. The title informs us

that have upgraded themselves "from a documentary to an attributive function." These, Chowdhury argues, are the ones we need to examine in Jibanananda's diction in order to transcend the "specificity of time [which] enlivens fictive figures, events and objects—renders them part of the daily journal; and translates imagination and thoughts into experience" (Chowdhury 2009). Just as the dandy's task of extracting the 'unchanging' from the 'transient' is case of a particular (and cultivated) form of gazing that is inextricably bound up the historically specific conditions of *la modernite*, Jibanananda's 'historic consciousness' filters the extent to which 'particular' histories affect the larger destiny of the human race. The world is apparent to the poet only in so far as it is 'lived' in this troubled decade, and not through some extended corridor that plays out an 'impossible' longing to go back to the villages of Bengal with their named, but ultimately imagined women (Arunima Sanyal, Suranjana, Banalata Sen or Mrinalini Ghoshal). In the poem 'Wristwatches,' a very specific 'temporal' event is abstracted to a generic understanding which leads up to a 'uniquely Jibananandian slant' on the real as the 'phosphorescent watch-faces of fallen soldiers' are brought out thus:

> "Their life's story will tick on a few moments more.
> Dim, and ever dimmer will they wake
> To the endless dark of sunlight, inexhaustible." (Seely 2006)

The oxymoron in the last line recalls familiar Miltonic and Shakespearean precedents. But to a large extent, it also connotes an epistemic confusion with regard to 'reading' the world order. This sense of befuddlement is a curious and historically specific characteristic identified by Walter Benjamin, for whom the shock induced by sensory bombardment in a city bustling with life ('*erlebnis*') and unmediated experience of it guaranteed by the constant mobility of the flaneur ('*erfahrung*') operate as the two opposing poles of a larger dialectic in an

that the suicide took place in the past. The poet is in the present recollecting a long past event. One can reasonably conclude that the poet has a sense of the past that works within his psyche"—Faizul Latif Chowdhury, Parabaas (URL given in the "References").

era of high capitalism (Benjamin 1983 (1935), 50). The fratricidal 'June Days' of 1848 were still not so distant in Baudelaire's memory, and feelings of shared despair and doubt-ridden class guilt are quite apparent in *Paris Spleen*. But this fact might also be rooted in the dandy's paradoxical projection of himself as an 'aristocrat' without the advantages of birth. Jibanananda on the other hand lived through a life of opposites—an unhappy marriage and the uncomfortable fact of his long unemployment might have helped him come to terms with the immediate, perceived reality of a life of hardship. For a man of Jibanananda's temperament, being an insurance agent for a private company in the 1940s can rightfully be called 'Sissyphean' and his 'rhetoric of walking' may well and truly have been informed by it.

IV: 'Imagined' Pathologies: The Metropolis and Mental Life

To what extent did the experience of the metropolis radically alter the 'mental life' of the man of modernity? Or, if we must pose the question differently: which are the conditions which structure of the modern episteme that is at odds with pre-modern systems of thought? How can these insights be reconciled to the peculiarly 'metropolitan' experience, and further, what 'diseases' does it bring about in the self-determination of Man?

Before we answer these questions, it is essential to clarify that we are comparing two artists who embody a 'rhetorical ambivalence—the shape-shifting, protean nature of their registers allow smooth transgressions from the generic constraints of either 'poetry' or 'prose.' Jibanananda's late oeuvre consists of three novels he completed with almost lightning pace during the year 1948. These are *Jalpaihati* (April-May 1948), *Sutirtha* (May-June 1948) and *Malyabaan* (June 1948). It will be my endeavour to point out, within a fairly limited scope, how these novels initiate a different 'rhetoric of illness' which is not just metaphoric or conceptual. The constraints of brevity here have directed me towards the partly 'unsatisfactory' and faulty methodology of textual sampling. Yet, I presume, given the breadth and expanse of these novels, it would not be possible to do otherwise. Here, the biographical details of Jibanananda's life will be relevant in constructing certain 'ways of seeing,' to borrow a phrase from John Berger, that impel the narratorial consciousness to look at a new semantics of what constitutes an 'illness' in the 'modern' era.

A host of characters in these novels suffer from a variety of ailments that go untreated, often due to the lack of money or means. The materiality of illness is carried over to the level of constructing plots i.e., they become lasting tropes on which the 'action' of these novels are constructed. *Jalpaihati* tells the story of Nishith Sen, a part-time lecturer at a college in would-be East Pakistan (echoing Jibanananda's own experiences of teaching at B.M. College, Barisal upto 1946) who comes to Calcutta to find a means of sustenance as well as to find out his elder daughter Ranu, exiled to this living theatre of changing forms through communal violence and Hindu-Muslim riots that did not spare Nishith's native Jalpaihati. He is surrounded by several forms of affliction. The failing health of his wife Sumana and that of his younger daughter Bhanu, suffering from tuberculosis in a nondescript hospital at Uttarpara does not help his cause. His son, Hareet, once a worker for the Indian National Congress, has now realised the futility of constitutional means in the nationalist struggle and is seen re-orienting himself to Marxist ideology. While in the city, Nishith puts up at the house of his old friend, Jiten Dasgupta at Ballygunge, now a corporate employee in the colonial mercantile firm, Graham and Graham. The glaring disparity between their respective social positions is not only highlighted at every turn of the plot, it becomes an enduring leitmotif for a social malady that is often covered up by the rhetoric of scientific progress and over-reliance on a historical positivism. A similar impulse, as my earlier analysis has shown, also motivated the 'anti-bourgeois' character of *dandysme.*

Jibanananda's plots are often monotonous and repetitive, drawing on events and situations that are part-autobiographical, and partly a result of the unique synthesis of the urban experience that his eponymous protagonists carry out in their minds. The 'uniqueness' in their perception stems from a dissociation between heightened individualism that the metropolis allows its inhabitants and the "calculating exactness of practical life which has resulted from a money economy (corresponds) to the ideal of natural science, namely that of transforming the world into an arithmetical problem" (Simmel 2000). The 'functional specialization of man and his work' in modernity makes 'one individual incomparable to another, and each of them indispensable to the highest possible extent.' Yet, the positivistic charge that is so bound up with our idea of what constitutes the 'modern' cannot accommodate all individuals equally in its fold. In order to survive the metropolis, it is imperative that an attitude of 'blasé indifference' may persist towards the qualitative distinctions between things. As the German sociologist Georg Simmel surmises:

> "...the meaning and the value of the distinctions between things, and therewith of the things themselves, are experienced as meaningless. They appear to the blasé person in a homogeneous, flat and gray colour with no one of them worthy of being preferred to another. This psychic mood is the correct subjective reflection of a complete money economy to the extent that money takes the place of all the manifoldness of things and expresses all qualitative distinctions between them in the distinction of how much." (Simmel 2000, 2001)

Jibanananda's novels depict protagonists who are mostly unemployed but married and with children they cannot satisfactorily 'tend to.' Clad in round-neck sweaters and dhoti, they trudge along the streets of the metropolis, meeting other characters, constantly revising their self-awareness of the strange world around them (Sultana 2015). These are usually achieved through interior monologues, playful *double entedres* and circular conversations that challenge the conventions of the realist novel. Unlike the dandy, Jibanananda's protagonists embody a directness and immediacy of perception about the moral order of 'bourgeois' values. The collective weight of their intellectual realisations transcend the notion of 'class guilt' as observed in Baudelaire; they deal with the problem of the metropolis through a calm resignation that seem to go hand in hand with the author's distrust in the capability of a positivistic turn that has makes 'science' a new religion. Classical Marxism too subscribed to such positivism—a movement that consolidated the civilisational indices of our culture as a whole. Therefore, in a broader context of 'historicity,' Jibanananda underlines the relative failure of all revolutions, Marxist or otherwise (Das, *Jalpaihati,* 1948: 11, 67; *Sutirtha*, 1948: 150). Both *Jalpaihati* and *Malyabaan* have plots constructed on this basic foundational schema. The eponymous protagonists in these two novels belong to the lower middle class and reject 'progress' in no uncertain terms, they do so even when they are located, in the fictive space of what they *are not.* An apt example of this occurs in the epistemic void between Malyabaan and his wife, Utpala. Just as the poet himself was a part of a 'failed' conjugal experience with his wife Labanya, the 'psychological interior' of Malyabaan's life is seen to be at radical odds with the lifestyle of extravagance and consumption embodied by his wife (Das, *Malyabaan* 2000).

In a sense, *Sutirtha* mediates between, and complements the other two novels in a way that must have been unforeseen by the author himself. Firstly, the class character of the eponymous protagonist is altered; like Jiten Dasgupta in *Jalpaihati,* Sutirtha too is a corporate employee, but one who is sensitive to the plight of those 'others' who do not fit the bill for 'progress.' His chance encounter with a young pickpocket Haran (who tries to steal from him) towards the beginning of the narrative can be thought of as proleptic in the sense of a foreboding that overshadows his other chance encounters with people on the streets. The way the specifics of personal identity in this encounter are abstracted to a general disillusionment with 'modern progress' is revelatory. In the course of a long, winding monologue that follows this encounter, Sutirtha realises that,

> "Whether you succeed in your convoluted tracks of the 'modern' and the 'pre-modern' is entirely your business. Who are these souls, lost in the never-ending labyrinth of those sublimely 'sharp' and shadowy paths? No one? Not someone?" (Das, *Sutirtha* 2000 (1948), 628, my translation)

Sutirtha's meeting with his old classmate Madhumangal, now turned a barber in a North Kolkata saloon, serves as an epilogue to this realisation. This episode is marked by an impossible nostalgia to go back to a world of relative certitude, "in the long, winding sleep of a world thirty or thirty-five years old, free from the maladies of the here-and-now" (Das, Sutirtha 2000 (1948), self-translated). The impossibility of going back to such a world is now beyond doubt. Despite taking part in the exchange, Sutirtha can only come to Madhumangal as a 'customer,' and not as his long-lost friend (Das, *Sutirtha* 2000 (1948), 628-633).

Through Madhumangal's open avowal of the threat of 'a contagious, venereal disease' in the sharp edges of his razor, an 'imagined pathology' of the modern initiates and terminates itself in a vicious cycle. This 'pathology' is specific to Jibanananda's protagonists, but its co-ordinates are older, and traceable to older pathologies[2]. Most notably, the paradoxical fascination and disgust with the nature of the metropolis allows "eccentricity, absurdity, horror, and ecstasy" to seep into his notion of modern life. The co-ordinates of the condition of metropolitan 'melancholia' were connected to "a mental constellation of revolt" (Hadlock 2001-2002). Kristeva too understands this condition in the context of an originary loss in man's sense of integrity. The 'hero of modernity' inhabits a strange 'heterotopic' space of oxymoron, like Nerval's metaphor of "an imagined sun, bright and black at the same time" (Kristeva 1989, 13). We need only turn to our examination of Jibanananda's late poetry (in the previous section) to confirm our speculations regarding a possible claim of rhetorical conflation between the oeuvre of the two poets.

If indeed a shared 'rhetoric of illness' between Baudelaire and Jibanananda's late oeuvre can be traced back to the condition of the 'modern,' the question now remains whether these comparable forms of 'gazing' relocate and reclaim what can be thought of as the 'iterability' of

[2] The inventory of diseases in Jibanananda's novels is fascinating and diverse. These include syphilis, gonorrhoea, insomnia, tuberculosis, cholera, chicken pox, malnutrition and pleurisy. Unless used as metaphor, they usually affect the narrator-protagonist and/or his family. In a remarkable section in *Sutirtha*, a (Hindu) character recalls having saved himself from communal violence owing to a 'circumcised' penis, the result of a surgery he had gone through in order to cure phimosis.

historical contexts. "The iterability of the trace (unicity, identification and alteration in repetition) is the condition of historicity," wrote Derrida, "and this iterability is also what lets the traces continue to function in the absence of a general context" (Derrida 2003, 1992). In so far as this paper has tried to reveal, the textual 'marks' of modernity in Jibanananda and Baudelaire appear to be 'iterable' in the rhetoricity of forms that envisage our manifold, and contesting modernities. To say that such 'marks' are originally 'iterable' therefore, is also to say that they "divide and repeat themselves immediately" (Derrida 2003, 26) in an endless regression.

We may presume *that* constitutes the 'modern' in our analysis, and both Baudelaire and Jibanananda inhabit these shared forms of belonging.

References

Baudelaire, Charles. (1869) 1970. "The Eyes of the Poor." In: *Paris Spleen*, translated by Louise Varese, 52-53. New York: New Directions.

Baudlaire, Charles. (1863) 1965. *The Painter of Modern Life and Other Essays.* Edited by Jonathan Mayne. Translated by Jonathan Mayne. London: Phaidon Press.

Baudelaire, Charles.(1857) 1982. "The Ragpicker's Wine." In: *Les Fleurs du Mal*, translated by Richard Howard, 103. New Hampshire: David R. Godine.

Benjamin, Walter. (1935) 1983.*Charles Baudelaire: A Lyric Poet in the Era of High Capitalism.* London: New Left Books (Verso)

Bermann, Marshall. 1982. *All that is Solid Melts into Air: The Experience of Modernity*. New York: Verso.

Chowdhury, Faizul Latif. 2009. "Temporality in the Poetry of Jibanananda Das." *Parabaas*, September. Accessed January 29, 2017. http://www.parabaas.com/translation/database/translations/essays/faizul_jibananan da.html.

Das, Jibanananda. 2000. *Jalpaihati.* Dhaka: Gatidhara, 2000.

Das, Jibanananda. (1948) 2000. *Malyabaan.* Dhaka: Gatidhara.

Das, Jibanananda. "Night." In: *Jibanananda Das: 29 Poems*, translated by Clinton B Seely. PoemHunter.com: The World's Poetry Archive, 2012 (1948).

Das, Jibanananda. (1948) 2000. *Sutirtha*. In: *Jibanananda Das er Upanyas-Samagra (Collection of Novels by Jibanananda Das)*. Dhaka: Gatidhara.

Derrida, Jacques. (1992) 2003. "This Strange Institution called Literature": An interview with Jacques Derrida. Vol. II, In: *Deconstruction: Critical Concepts in Literary and Cultural Studies*, edited by Jonathan D Culler. London and New York: Routledge.

Foucault, Michel. 1984. "What is Enlightenment?" In: *The Foucault Reader*, by Michel Foucault, edited by Paul Rabinow. New York: Patheon Books.

Hadlock, Philip G.2001-02. "The 'Other' Other: Baudelaire, Melancholia, and the Dandy." *Nineteenth-Century French Studies* 30. 1/2 (Fall-Winter): 58.

Herman, Arthur. 2009. *Gandhi and Churchill: The Epic Rivalry that Destroyed an Empire and Forged Our Age*. New York: Bantam Books.

Knepler, Henry, ed. *Man About Paris: The Confessions of Arsene Houssaye*. London: Victor Gollancz Ltd, 1972.

Kristeva, Julia. *Black Sun: Depression and Melancholia*. New York: Columbia UP, 1989.

Mukhopadhyay, Sanjay. 2011. "Harrison Road ey aro Gobheer Awsukh (Deeper Maladies on Harrison Road)." *Parabaas*. Accessed January 26, 2016. http://www.parabaas.com/jd/articles/pSanjay1.shtml.

Seely, Clinton B. 2006. "The Scent of Sunlight : Poems by Jibanananda Das." *Parabaas*. Accessed January 26, 2016. http://parabaas.com/jd/articles/seely_scent.shtml.

Seigel, Jerrold. 1986. *Bohemian Paris: Culture, Politics, and the Boundaries of Bourgeois Life*, 1830-1930. New York: Elizabeth Sifton Books.

Simmel, Georg. 2000. "The Metropolis and Mental Life." In: *The City Cultures Reader*, edited by Malcom Miles, Tim Hall and Borden Iain, 1999-2005. New York: Routledge.

Sultana, F. 2015. "Jibanananda Das er Upyanyase Astitver Sankate Manush (The Crisis of Human Identity in the Novels of Jibanananda Das)." *Jibanananda Das Rachanabali.* http://jibonanondo-rachanaboli.info/.

Wheatcroft, Geoffrey. 2015. "Review of *Churchill and Empire* by Lawrence James." *The New York Times*, August 15. Accessed January 29, 2017. https://www.nytimes.com/2014/08/17/books/review/churchill-and-empire-by-lawrence-james.html?_r=0.

Part 2.
Literature, Medicine and Healthcare in Colonial India

In: Imperial Maladies
Editors: D. Bandyopadhyay et al.
ISBN: 978-1-53611-863-6

Chapter 4

INDIAN PERSPECTIVES OF MEDICINE AND THE COLONIAL ERA

Chaitali Maitra*
Department of English, St. Paul's Cathedral Mission College,
Kolkata, West Bengal, India

The most happening period in human history was making itself felt in every possible way: everywhere there was more and more experimentation leading to more and more discoveries that marked the late nineteenth century and the beginning of the twentieth century. Every new vista opened had a new promise. This was particularly true of medicine. The new generation of scientists had known and studied the humoural theory; but now they had to understand the germ theory of disease. As a result, there was a sea-change in the perception and the diagnosis of the rampant diseases of these times. As Tony Farmar points out:

*Author's Address: Dept. of English, St. Paul's Cathedral Mission College, 33/1, Raja Rammohan Roy Road, Baithakkhana, Kolkata, West Bengal, India. PIN: 700006, Email: chaitalisubrata@hotmail.com.

> The new theory finally rendered obsolete debility and miasma and a thousand other terms of art. . . . Initially the medical profession had great difficulty in discarding the ancient wisdom that diseases were always multi-caused. (Farmar 2004,101)

As the physicians struggled to incorporate the new and the old at a meeting in 1905 of the State Medicine Section of the Royal Academy of Medicine of Ireland, the president of the college, Sir John Moore presented a paper linking the rise in soil temperature to the incidence of mortality from diarrhoea; after much debate Dr. James Craig, a later president too, observed that this terrible disease was caused by micro-organisms. The great medical textbook by William Osler 'Principles and Practice of Medicine' published in 1892, took a lot of time to run into editions, establishing the organisms of typhoid and tuberculosis.

With more and more information on the nature of the diseases, and the treatment that could be offered, the absolute divide between medicine and surgery decreased. By the middle of the 19th century both these strands were learning to thrive together. Anaesthesia was becoming established, the antibiotics discovered, the stethoscope becoming a hallmark for a doctor (Udwadia 2000, 299). Collateral to this, the same decades had been more heroic in the Irish medicine. The Irish school of clinicians made names like Robert Graves, Dominic Corrigan and William Stokes (for a special disease, pulse and heart-block respectively), become celebrities which also made them famous overseas (Woods 1982,44). With such brilliant insights, more challenging operations could be performed. The novelist Charles Lever, who was also a doctor, had his tooth removed with ether and was immensely thankful for the lessening of pain; he prophesied that this would have a great impact in the social life of the people who were in the two minds about the quality of relief, anaesthesia could give.

Medicine in colonial India and its subsequent development, however, had a different history. Far from being just the case of an innocent philanthropic enterprise, it was also closely linked to the socio-economic policies of segregation and dominance practised by the existing colonial power as well as native elites in India. The advent of Western healthcare facilities in the Indian domains were a product of wars over economic, imperialist, and mercantile concerns between contending factions which directly implied that the common populace being of indirect and trivial consequence to the administrators often fell out of the purview of the aforementioned facilities. A probe into the origins of medical facilities in colonial India would affirm a limited, regional character of the initial establishments founded to cater to the needs of the soldiers involved in inter-territorial wars against the French, Mysore, or Maratha confederacies. This is substantiated by the fact that hospitals in the presidency towns such as Royal Naval Hospital at Madras, Medical College and Hospital at Calcutta catered largely to the British and Indian troops involved in the wars. Such hospitals were indispensable owing to the rise in tropical diseases amongst the Company troops, thereby multiplying the mortality rate among the recruits. In due time, the surgeons from Britian, primarily Irish and Scottish, employed in the hospitals extended their services to the Indians who were able to afford it despite religious or cultural concerns.

Apart from setting up hospitals for the treatment of war injuries and tropical diseases in soldiers, the foundations of a Lunatic Asylum was laid in Monghyr in 1795 for the confinement of the insane, on the lines of similar institutions in Georgian England. The enterprise though short lived reflected hegemonic concerns on Foucauldian terms. The primary function of the Lunatic Asylum was disciplinary that entailed the maintenance of order by eliminating any symptom of defiance to the reigning authority. Additionally, these spaces served as grounds for the isolation of sepoys after contracting venereal diseases as has been observed by Seema Alavi in her work *The Sepoys and the Company: Tradition and Transition in Northern India* (Alavi 1995). The fact that the objectives of healthcare as provided by the Company were solely directed towards the well being of the sepoys can be judged by the fact that special "lock hospitals" were created for the treatment of the prostitutes serving the sepoys for the prevention of sexually transmitted diseases. This fact has been fictionally presented by Amitav Ghosh in his third book of the Ibis Trilogy, *Flood of Fire* (2015), where he narrates multiple liasions of sepoys stationed at Calcutta with local prostitutes leading to "unspeakable" diseases.

It took a considerable amount of time for the institutionalized healthcare to include the civilian populace in the ambit of its benefits; for the Company seeking to intensify territorial hold was seldom interested in interfering with the populace which was beset by bouts of Asiatic cholera, malaria, leprosy, anthrax, influenza, tuberculosis and so on which often assuming the proportions of pandemic were responsible in wiping considerable portions of the native population from time to time. The aforesaid diseases formed the plot of several creations of regional Indian literature, for instance in the works of Fakirmohan Senapati, Gopinath Mohanty, or Phanishwar Nath Renu. In Senapati's 'Rebati', Asiatic cholera appearing as an epidemic caused the deaths of Rebati's parents and later the only living benefactor, the village schoolmaster. Later in the story, the eponymous protagonist's fate is also sealed in the similar fashion by the same incurable disease. Gopinath Mohanty's *Paraja* narrates the tale of tribes, the Parajas and their closed economy confined within the realms of the forest of Koraput region in Orissa. It can be seen that the natives being better equipped with negotiating the tough living conditions empathise with the failing physique of the young White officer posted in their region who loses his life to Malaria in the absence of western and indigenous treatments.

A more complex narrative forms the structure of Phanishwar Nath Renu's 'Maila Aanchal' where following the journey of Prashant Banerjee or Doctor Babu of Maryganj in Purnea, one becomes aware of the extraneous factors having extensive bearings on the reluctance of the Company towards the provision of a democratic healthcare service. As can be gathered from the progression of the plot, facilitating communal healthcare mechanism was further complicated by several factors such as the expanse of administrative territory, presence of diverse ethnic groups, prevalence of economic and caste based distinctions, and interrelated religious and cultural beliefs. These issues have been adequately explored by David Arnold in his work *Science, Technology, and Medicine in Colonial India* where he observes that caste based cultural segregations were so deep rooted that the practitioners of Western medicine were subjected to distrust to an extent that inoculation and vaccination measures were on the verge of retrenchment. However, in due course, says Arnold, "Medicine lifted the veil of purdah 'without irreverence'; it broke down the barriers of caste 'without sacrilege'. Medical science was 'the most cosmopolitan of all sciences' because it embraced 'in its merciful appeal every suffering human being in the world'" (Arnold 2004, 137). The distrust arose as a result of the discourse of distancing entailed by the practice of western colonial medicine dominating the scene of nineteenth century Bengali theatre. The plays enacted with colonial medicine and its practitioners as subjects were either satiric (prahasan) in tone or in the darpan mode attempting to lay bare certain truths for the public. Most of these plays in the initial days such as Rajkrishna Roy's 'Daktarbabu' or Dr. Sundarimohan Das' *Munisipal Darpan* (1892), especially of the satiric mode depicted the doctor as a distanced, unmoved entity placed a level higher than the regular countrymen lacking empathy or fraternal concern for their less privileged counterparts. The doctors found in Kamakhyaprasad Roy's 'Mayapuri'(1937) or Sachindranath Sengupta's 'Narsin Home'(1940) were presented as adherents of excessive commercialisation, sexual and moral corruption, and excessive monetary concerns thereby exposing the moral degeneration unleashed by the proliferation of the discourses of the masters.

This scene was transformed post 1920 with the arrival of texts on the literary scene that popularised the image of a doctor governed by public welfare concerns. An instance of the same can be seen in the portrayal of Dr. Agniswar Mukherji in Banaphool's novel *Agniswar* (immortalised in the film 'Agniswar' by Uttam Kumar) where the fictional character is depicted to be a strict professional true to his ethics. Underneath that callous exterior was a doctor combating the medical corruption and empathising with the human condition by making secret donations to improve the living conditions of the underprivileged in the region, always prioritising the humanitarian concerns.

The cause for slow pace of the progress of healthcare amongst the populace can be attributed to the lack of state sponsors. In its primary stages, healthcare was largely dependent on private subscriptions, as can be seen in the case of the failed proposal of Calcutta Fever Hospital in 1836, the establishment of which was supposed to be funded by Europeans and affluent Indian population. The administration with its mercantile mindsetwas disinclined to mobilise funds towards healthcare or another inextricably linked issue – sanitation. Such measures though vital were delegated to the purview of respective municipal councils which proved unsuccessful in raising adequate funds to achieve the goals of providing even the basic sanitation to the region under its jurisdiction. Additionally, the public unrest caused by the instatement of a property tax in Benares in 1810 prevented any further iteration of the model in other provincial towns. It was the personal initiatives of the Governor Generals of India Lord Wellesley and Lord Bentinck that sanitation was undertaken as principal concern but only in certain privileged portions of the respective cities. Under the former, in 1803 the excessive vegetation around the town and the expansive salt lake to the east of Calcutta was cleared with the proposal for instating a working drainage system. Lord Bentinck, during his office had proposed for a full fledged sanitary system which remained unrealised owing to the meagre revenue raised by municipal authorities. Vaccination and inoculation against tropical diseases like small pox also witnessed a slow progress in India despite the establishment of a working Indian Medical Service in the mid-eighteenth century. Such measures were undertaken by the provincial administration directly to enhance the popularity of the non-native government among the masses. Often adjudged on economic terms, it was believed that every life saved was additional revenue and an increase to the population and the prosperity of the Company's territories in an incalculable ratio.

It should not be assumed that the history of western medicine in colonial India is a straightforward chronicle of introduction and assimilation for the discourse and subsequent practice as a cultural phenomenon underwent a rigorous process of acculturation characterised by intricate web of hybridisation. It is a polysemic discourse involving cultural, spatial, and economic concerns in the classification of diseases and in extension, the natives victimised by the same. The class concerns were evident in the statute governing the admissions of students to Calcutta Medical College which stated that all native youths between the age of fourteen and twenty with respectable family connections shall be eligible for admission to the college. This resulted in the first batch of graduates belonging to the topmost layers of the native class hierarchy in Bengal being recruited as Sub-Assistant Surgeons despite the demand of higher salaries than their lower class counterparts who were absorbed as dressers and compounders owing to their class affiliations. On similar lines, Dr. Lakshmikanta Ali observed that diseases like Dropsy and Beriberi were more common amongst poor Muslims living in huts with earthen roof tiles under the absence of basic sanitation (Ali 1909, 329). Another observation was presented by Dr. Lalmohan Ghoshal of Rajshahi Government Hospital that Bengalis were more affected by malaria or Bengal fever affected than the Europeans, adding that the aforesaid ailment targeted villagers more than urban residents and the poor more than the genteel. (Ghosal 1906, 245) Examples abound in the novels of Sarat Chandra Chattopadhyay and also Tara Shankar Bandyopadhyay. In the novel, *BirajBou*, Biraj talks of 'malori' (meaning malaria) as something very common in the neighbourhood. Plague is presented as death incarnate in novels like *Grihadaha*, where Ramesh throws himself to nurse the sick and infected plague patients.

In spite of spelling loyalty to western medical practices, the native surgeons failed to shed the influences of the indigenous medical systems which were explicit in their response to diagnosis of diseases and suggested measures for prevention and control. In one of his articles titled "Bangali Saheb Nahe", the medical scholar D. D. Gupta established the anatomical differences that characterise the physique of the Bengalis and Europeans, proclaiming that the "Bengalis were not Englishmen" (Gupta 1901) and the difference in constitution made the former more susceptible to contagions and epidemics. Cholera, as an epidemic was also first found in Bengal, amounting to innumerable deaths due to lack of awareness and medicine.

Thus, there was an immediate need of a set of curative practices, differing in approach from western colonial modes of treatment, dedicated to understanding the Bengali constitution and administering relevant treatment. Further contribution in this direction was made by Devendranath

Roy and Dr. Satyasaran Chakrabarty who propounded a germ theory of diseases according to which infectious disease were caused owing to the lack of vital life force in each cell constituting the physical frame of the human in question. On the lines of Ayurveda, preference was given to sanguine, phlegmatic, bilious, nervous temperaments of human beings that existing either alone or in combinations called for different modes of treatment. A more cogent example can be traced in the text of Gunga Persaud Mookerjee (*The Principles and Practice of Medicine in Bengali*) where he asserts that light-skinned, blue-eyed, thick-haired men possessing a combination of contradictory temperaments were more prone to tuberculosis and scrofula than their counterparts. (Mookerjee 1877, 8) Following, similar tenets, gunas or primal qualities of a person were used by Dr. Harimohan Sen to adjudge his susceptibility to contagion (Sen 1911, 420). The inferences drawn by the aforesaid practitioners were undoubtedly based on keen observation and painstaking analysis of facts. This however, has to be understood that the factors enumerated above are extraneous to the domain of western medicine and reflect crucial instances of a troubled creolisation of an otherwise objective, desensitised body of cultural practices.

The history of colonial medicine, in extension can be read as a chronicle of the assimilation of Western discursive practices in the otherwise impregnable opacity of Indian cultural practices. The progression from the dominant indigenous modes of treatment encompassing nature, namely Ayurveda, Unani, and a confounding gamut of religious practices to adopting Western medicine reflects an interconnected renaissance in the system of Indian history of ideas (Roy 1986). This trend can be observed in Tarasankar Bandopadhyay's *Arogya Niketan* where the transition from the old medicinal practices to the systematised Western modes of treating illness and the conflicting intricacies are brought to the fore. The transition from the modes of Jibon Mashai to Pradyut apart from exposing a shift in trends of reception towards healthcare also reflects a tilt towards materialist culture of the colonial administrators. The novel displays a transition in the perceived attitude towards death from an interlude in the cycle of eternal life to ultimate cessation of the process of life. Jibon Mashai decided to stop seeing patients after the death of Bonbihari; and later when he was trying to examine the pulse of Miya Syed Abu Taher, remembered the dying moments of Manjari, whom he loved to distraction. The same insight is also seen in 'Agradaani' of Tara Shankar Bandopadhyay and *Putulnacher Itikatha* (1935) of Manik Bandopadhyay. For Bandopadhyay, reaching out to the rather lower classes of Rarh Bangla, becomes a matter of conscience which has an embedded sense of echo in his past. In fact, *Arogya Niketan* also shows how the marginalised also find their meagre healthcare, more often in the kabiraj-hakim ethos. In this novel where relationships are weighed against so many absolutes Jibon Mashai's attitude to death definitely determines the Indian attitude. In one of the passages in the novel one reads about the early morning rays of the sun falling on a young palm leaf – this can be used to heal the sick. Also, the hidden part of the leaf which has not been exposed to daylight could be boiled to use the vapour to decrease pain. Jibon Mashai's respect for 'mustiyoga' that he learned from his father through his grandfather, who had learned the same from a monk (Bandyopadhyay (1953) 1975, 109). The stance is far removed from the 'modern' medicine but the novelist's forte is neither the old nor the new medicine; he is trying to delve deep into the belief system which tries to look at the natural-primordial nexus. To this, the modern medicine comes with a promise of cure; but this, unknowingly and often, belittles the human aspect of treating the less privileged and the sick.

The works of these writers would further establish the fact that healthcare and medical facilities as offered by the colonial masters also served to be an instrument for securing unwavering consent of the masses for its administrative and colonial facilities. Dropped mortality rates and a marked improvement in the quality of life would mean the erasure of the subtlest forms of rebellion and an adherence to the culture of the masters, thereby securing their rule for a considerable period of time. Most regional literature of these times tried to establish the importance of the humanitarian perspective, thereby establishing a subtle controversy evident in the apparent master list of success and the sordid reality of the lives of the colonised. This also raises the central question about the human values in the Indian ethos, asking the pertinent question of how to lead life and the best way to evaluate it.

REFERENCES

Alavi, Seema. 1995. *The Sepoys and the Company: Tradition and Transition in Northern India, 1770-1830*. Delhi: Oxford University Press.

Ali, Laksmikanta. 1909. "Epidemic Dropsy ba Sankramak Shoth". *Bhishak Darpan*, 19.9: 328-35.

Arnold, David. 2004. The New Cambridge History of India: *Science, Technology and Medicine in Colonial India.* Cambridge: Cambridge University Press.

Banaphool. 1989. Agniswar. In *Banaphool Granthavali*. Kolkata: Granthalaya.

Bandyopadhyay, Tarashankar. 1975. ArogyaNiketan. In *Tarashankar Rachanavali*, vol. 10. 3-310. Kolkata: Mitra O Ghosh.

Chattopadhyay, Saratchandra. 1976. Grihadaha. In *Sarat Rachanavali.* 231-400. Kolkata: Sarat Samiti.

Das, Sundarimohan. 1892. *Municipal Darpan* (*The Municipal Mirror*). Kolkata: Prabhakar Yantra.

Farmar, Tony. 2004. *Patients, Potions and Physicians*. Dublin: A and A Farmar.

Ghosal, Lalmohan. 1906. "Banglar Jwar Sammandhe Mantabya" ("Opinions on Fever in Bengal"). *Bhishak Darpan*, 16.7: 245-47.

Gupta, D.D. 1901. "Bangali Saheb Nahe" ("Bengalis are not Englishmen"). *Swasthya* 5.2: 36-37.

Mookerjee, Gunga Persaud. 1877. *The Principles and Practice of Medicine in Bengali*. Calcutta: Saptahik Sambad Press.

Ray, Binoy Bhusan. 1986. *Chikitsha Bigganer Itihaas*. (History of Medicine) Kolkata: Patraput.

Sen, Harimohan. 1911. 'Swasthya Raksa o Swasthya Unnatir Upaya.' ("Preservation of Health and Ways of Improving Health") *Bhisak Darpan* 21, 11 and 12: 401-28.

Udwadia, Farokh Erach. 2000. *Man and Medicine*, Oxford: Oxford University Press.

Woods, J. O. 1982. "The History of Medicine in Ireland." *Ulster Medical Journal* 51.1: 35–45.

In: Imperial Maladies
Editors: D. Bandyopadhyay et al.
ISBN: 978-1-53611-863-6

Chapter 5

DISEASES AND HEALTHCARE IN KIPLING'S SHORT STORIES

Abidita Goswami*
Department of English, Budge Budge College,
Kolkata, West Bengal, India

> Fever is the great scourge and calamity of India, for natives as well as Europeans. (Beattie 2011, 39)
>
> – Dietrich Brandis, 1833.

The establishment of imperialism on tropical lands had adverse effects not only on the colonised but also on the colonisers. The inability of the Europeans to adjust to the tropical climate was, initially, not thought of. It threatened to weaken their imperial grip over colonized countries. In tropical countries like India, European soldiers suffered greatly from diseases leading to death or invalidity. The uprisings of 1857 added to the health anxieties of imperial policy makers. Hence, various measures were

---

*Corresponding Author's Email: abiditaagoswami@gmail.com.

designed to improve the health conditions of the English troops. Although better nutrition and clothing and clean drinking water were provided to the soldiers, the risk of famines and disease outbreaks continued to maintain imperial anxieties. The need to maintain a healthy and strong military force in order to continue dominance, led to medical legislations, discoveries in medical fields and environmental modifications.

With the rise of microbial science, the focus shifted from environment to humans. Everyone belonging to the tropics, irrespective of their classes, was considered to be a carrier of diseases. The efforts to improve medicines and increased supply of medical help in India were mainly to protect the health of the colonialists living in India. The imperialists were forced to live in alien lands in order to maintain their dominance, as a result of which they suffered greatly from the diseases contracted from the colonized mass. Outbreak of diseases like cholera and typhoid took away lives of several men, women and children from both ends of the colonial system. As a result, medical help was sent to the tropical lands to cure the colonised people as it was from them that the imperialists contracted the diseases. This was often disguised as a modest attempt to serve the plague-stricken and diseased colonised people who are in dire need of help.

The association of Indians with diseases became a commonly considered fact, and the outbreak of diseases in India along with the attempt of the Europeans to heal them, formed a basis of several works in literature. Joseph Rudyard Kipling's literary works on India are full of references to medicines and diseases. Diseases like plague, influenza, cholera and the like form an indispensable part of Kipling's short stories as well as his poetry and novels. Not only the diseases but also the efforts to eradicate them, the medical initiatives taken by the Europeans, can be found in his works. Born in India, Kipling viewed the country through the eyes of the European person who knew the place better than England. The comfort with which he wrote about India shows his relations to the land. Being a European and at the same time, being born in India, Kipling could clearly perceive the effects of colonialism on the coloniser as well as on the colonised.

In most of his short stories, Kipling talked about the outbreak of diseases in various parts of India and how the Europeans contracted the same when they tried to serve the diseased. Though the themes of the stories are diverse, the base is always founded on tropical diseases. 'By Word of Mouth' is one of the finest short stories of Kipling that deal with the outbreak of typhoid and cholera. Based on a paranormal theme, the story gives an account of the life of Dumoise, a Civil Surgeon and how his wife and Dumoise himself fall prey to the epidemic. The story indicates how imperialism had adverse effects on the imperialist himself. The feeling of living on a land that is completely different from the home atmosphere is revealed when Kipling says, "Few people can afford to play Robinson Crusoe anywhere – least of all in India, where we are few in the land, and very much depended on each other's kind offices" (Kipling 1884, 14). Kipling's keen interest in the medical field can be understood in his vivid descriptions of disease outbreaks and the remedial steps taken to cure them. "Nearly every household in India knows that Doctors are very helpless in typhoid. The Battle must be fought between Death and the Nurses, minute by minute and degree by degree" (Kipling 1884, 21). The reactions of the characters like Mrs. Shute and others and also their knowledge about the epidemics show the frequency of diseases and the inevitablity of the consequences suffered by the Europeans for living in close proximity to the epidemic.

Death by tropical diseases was a well-known and accepted fact for the Europeans. Hence, when Dumoise receives the telegram from Shimla, ordering him to go to Nuddea to serve the people suffering from the outbreak of cholera, he knew that it was his end. Although Kipling has portrayed the incidents through a paranormal lens focusing on the spirit of his deceased wife, the sense of helplessness and inevitable death due to the diseases can be clearly understood through the character of Ram Dass. Ram Dass claims to have seen the spirit of his Memsahib who has sent a message for Dumoise through him that she would meet him in Nuddea. This message indicates the impending death of Dumoise in Nuddea. But the Memsahib does not mention anything about the life of Ram Dass. Yet he fears that if he accompanies his master to Nuddea, he might lose his own life. "He was not going to Nuddea to see his Sahib die, and, perhaps to die himself" (Kipling 1884, 22).

Moreover, the story also portrays how the death of a doctor while trying to save lives was quite natural. When Dumoise dies of cholera after eleven days of service in Nuddea, he is quickly replaced by a "fresh doctor" who could continue his service of coping with the epidemic. Hence, the very fact that Dumoise is a surgeon makes his death and suffering quite natural and inevitable. He is one among the many doctors who sacrifice their lives trying to serve the people. Though the character of Dumoise is brilliantly depicted the complete focus on the life of the surgeon brings out the Eurocentric tendencies of the literary works. Throughout the story, the focus never shifts to the colonised people suffering from the epidemic. Nor is there any account of the number of deaths or how the Indians become a prey to the outbreak of cholera and typhoid.

Kipling's narratives often bring out the inability to build some absolute ground for the cause of empire or for his *de jure* homeland India. In terms of diseases, he sympathises with the imperialists dying helplessly in India but also indicates it to be the result of their own actions. It is the urge to continue dominance over the tropical lands for which more and more Europeans were sent to India. The increased anxieties of the imperialists in relation to tropical diseases have also been brought out by Kipling, quite comically, in his works. One of the finest examples is his short story, 'A Germ Destroyer'.

First published in the *Civil and Military Gazette* on May 17, 1887, and then, in the first edition of *Plain Tales from the Hills* in 1888, the story points out farcically the downside of the administrative world of the British Raj. The eccentricity of E. S. Mellish, the inventor, clearly indicates the desperation of the imperialists to save their people living on the colonized land. Mellish's invention of the fumigatory powder to kill cholera germs after a research of fifteen years indicates the attempts to invent colonial medicines to be used in countries like India. Kipling brilliantly brings out the humour in the actions of the inventor as well as in the actions of the Viceroy. The maintainence of the Indian Empire had grown difficult day by day due to the invalidity of the officials who were sent to administer India. The frequency of diseases made the European troops weak for which they could not suppress the Indian rebels with a strong hand. This increased the pressure on the imperialists to invent new medicines for India.

The very title of the story brings out the farce contained in it and also its central focus. Kipling has given an ironical justification to the title as, at the end, Mellish is successful in destroying the germ, that is, the Private Secretary, John Fennil Wonder. The Viceroy is finally relieved from the over-officious Wonder who used to "draw matters which were entirely outside his province into his own hands." (Kipling 2016, 65). Although the story takes a different turn, 'A Germ Destroyer', just like 'By Word of Mouth', is founded on disease and its cure. The fact that the Viceroy gets amused by the inventor who does not talk "shop" (Kipling 2016, 64) like the missed out guest, E. Mellish, represents the increased interest of the Europeans living in India about the prevention of the diseases. Even when the Viceroy realises that Mellish is not the actual guest of the day, he still seems to be impressed by him as he thinks, "Evidently, this is the wrong tiger; but it is an original animal" (Kipling 2016, 65). When the monomaniac inventor fumigates the room to kill cholera germs, the Viceroy still seems to be amused at his actions though he is almost choked to death due to the thick black smoke. The irony is maintained when Kipling mentions that Wonder resigns from his position on "health grounds" (Kipling 2016, 66) while actually it was due to the allegations of the Viceroy.

Besides the farcical actions of Mellish and the other characters, the story does not fail to bring out Kipling's brilliance in describing diseases and their cure, the latter being original or fictitious. Through the inferences drawn by the inventor, Kipling talks vividly about the disease, Cholera. "He held that cholera was a germ that propagated itself as it flew through a muggy atmosphere; and stuck in the branches of trees like a wool-flake. The germ could be rendered sterile, he said, by 'Mellish's Own Invincible Fumigatory'- a heavy violent-black powder- 'the result of fifteen years' scientific investigation, Sir!'" (Kipling 2016, 66).

Kipling had a special interest in medicine, which is evident not only in his description of diseases and their treatment, but also in the portrayal of the characters of Doctors and Inventors of medicine. He was greatly influenced by physicians and inventors since a very young age, and throughout his life, he has written several stories, poems and novels describing their lives and works. In 1909, Kipling wrote a story based on the life of Nicholas Culpeper. He had acquired a copy of his book on Herbals which became the basis of his short story 'A Doctor of Medicine'. He was also influenced by Rene Laennec, the inventor of the stethoscope, the reflections of which can be found in his work, 'Marklake Witches'. Even the American setting in his adventure story 'Captain Courageous' is created with the help of his close friend, James Conland who was his personal physician. In one of his popular poems, 'If', he has given a tribute to his physician friend, Leandar Starr Jameson, who was associated with the Boer War and later became the Prime Minister of the Cape Colony. Hence, Kipling never failed to make the issues concerning diseases and medical health a very important and integral part of his stories.

Often as it has been witnessed, the rejection of colonialism by the Indians and other colonised countries often led to rejection of every object introduced by the colonists, however useful it might have proved for them. This was clearly visible in case of the medicines introduced by the Europeans in the colonised lands. Journals like *Oudh Akhbar* which was published in Lucknow claimed that Unani was at par with the European medicines and rejected the latter on the basis of the fact that they were not rooted in the Indian locale. Moreover, the movements against imperialism included a search for Indian identity. As a result, traditional medicines, most importantly Ayurveda became an integral part of their rebellion. Several colleges, pharmaceutical industries and practices of Ayurveda and Unani medicines became popular during the British Raj. The introduction of Western medicines led rise to indigenous therapeutics and increased the efforts to find indigenous alternatives to European pharmaceuticals. Moreover, the expensiveness of the Western medicines convinced Western-trained Indian doctors like S. S. Sokhey and R. N. Chopra to find cheaper and easily accessible indigenous drugs.

Even though intensive research was being conducted by European and Indian doctors, the frequency of famines and epidemics were beyond control. India, being a tropical country is dependent on monsoon rains and hence, it often faces crop failures and is hit by famines. The frequency has reduced to a considerable extent in the modern times but the situation was at its worse during the British rule in India. The British Government failed to settle a famine policy till 1866. Staying in India for a while led Kipling to witness a number of famine outbreaks. He had seen people suffering and dying in thousands. He had also witnessed how relief was sent from Europe and how Europeans shared the plight of the natives in India. An elaborate description of the same can be studied in another short story by Kipling, titled 'William the Conqueror'.

Based on the experiences of two Anglo-Indian relief workers during their service in famine-stricken British India, 'William the Conqueror' remains an invaluable document portraying the imperialist and humanitarian missions of the British Raj. The story had initially faced critical oblivion, but it was through the work of Wallace Ruddell concerning the history of famine and twentieth century famine relief that the short story was rescued. The story appeared in two parts, in December 1895 in *The Gentlewoman* (England) and later in January 1896 in *The Ladies' Home Journal* (USA). It was then collected in *The Days' Work* in 1898. The plot of the story has been rightly expressed by Kipling himself in a letter to Mr. Edward Bok, a friend of Kipling as well as the author and publisher of *The Ladies' Home Journal*, "…It deals with a wooing in the thick of a Madras famine- man and girl together working hard among the starving and feeding the abandoned black babies and generally going through deep waters: and it ends with their joyful return to their home province, the Punjab, in time for the festivities of the 'Christmas week.'" (Pinney 1990, 176).

William the Conqueror undoubtedly describes the famine-stricken India in the most vivid manner, but it also positions Kipling absurdly, both as a mouthpiece of imperialism who tries desperately to justify the ways of colonialism in India and at the same time, portraying the impossible pretensions of imperialism. The very title of the story associates the entire plot with a "conquest" or colonialism. Even though Scott works selflessly to provide relief to the perishing babies and the sufferers in South India, the ultimate attitude of the relief workers towards him becomes an example of what Gayatri Chakraborty Spivak calls "benevolent imperialism" (Kuokkanen 2007, 82). The story throws light upon the Anglo-Indian community, people who consider themselves to be a part of India, but still feel alienated amidst situations of dire sufferings. It also marks the differences of the southern and northern regions of the country as the Anglo Indians, living in the northern parts for years together, suddenly end up feeling alienated in the South, about which they have no knowledge. "Then the languages in which the names of the stations were written changed, and they launched south into a foreign land, where the very smells were new" (Kipling 2015, 81).

The story provides several contrasting ideas reflected by Kipling against the background of tropical diseases and healthcare. On one hand, Kipling points out the varied lifestyles of the people in different parts of India. When Scott finds out that the grains they have brought from the northern regions, that is, wheat, millet and barley are rejected by the people of the South who would eat only rice, it marks the differences between the food habits of two regions of the same country. At the same time, Kipling is found to have often generalised the mass under one title, "subalterns" or the children as "black babies" (Kipling 2015, 82). Similarly, the portrayal of the Anglo-Indians show certain discrepancies, when on the one hand, they identify themselves as a part of the Indian region in which they live, and on the other hand, distinguish themselves from the Other. On one side we find Mrs. Jim telling William, "You're a Punjabi, too, you know." (Kipling 2015, 82). Even towards the end of the second part, when William feels relieved to have reached the northern regions and feels homely in the midst of her own people, it brings out the deep relations that the colonialists were building due to their close associations with the natives. But at the same time, we find a continuous reference to white men and their difference from the natives. The sharp contrast between Faiz Ullah and Scott and the attitude of the former towards the latter bring out the irremovable sense of a master-slave relationship between the coloniser and the colonised. When Faiz Ullah tells Martyn's servant, "Thou and I, O brother, will thus secure the servants' places close by; and because of our masters' authority none will dare to disturb us" (Kipling 2015, 83), he completely acknowledges the supreme authority of the imperialists.

The contradiction is most visible in case of William. William represents the story's feminised hero, a classic warrior who has fought and survived for four years since her coming to India. "Twice she had been nearly drowned while fording a river; once she had been run away with on a camel; had witnessed a midnight attack of thieves on her brother's camp; had seen justice administered, with long sticks, in the open under trees"(Kipling 2015, 84). Like a typical colonialist falling a prey to the tropical diseases, she "had been through a very bad cholera year, seeing sights unfit to be told; and had wound up her experiences by six weeks of typhoid fever." (Kipling 2015, 85). But, unlike the soldiers or other Europeans who died or remained invalid, she got back to her feet and actively participated with his brother Martyn in the service of the diseased. Towards the end of the story, Lord Jim acknowledges her as a stronger person than her brother Martyn. Yet, throughout the story, she carries the identity of a weaker sex, who strives to acquire a male personality in order to break through the limitations of the feminine world. Giving up the habit of writing letters to her aunts or cutting the pages of the English magazines and cropping her hair as well as her name short, that is, from Wilhelmina to William, she tries to come out of the image of a stereotype Victorian woman.

The situation of famine adds to the subject of masculine colonial dominance in the story when Scott clearly states, "A famine's no place for a woman" (Kipling 2015, 84). Kipling points out how unusual it was of a woman participating in a famine relief act, through the words of Scott, "There aren't many women, sisters or wives, who would walk into a famine with their eyes open" (Kipling 2015, 85). Inspite of her struggle to rise above the notion of a delicate woman and trying to come out as a true hero, she fails to attain utmost importance in the story. Though the title of the story recalls her character, it is ultimately Scott who comes out as the hero and the saviour of the masses. While Scott engages himself in milking goats and feeding the babies, carrying carts full of grains and working selflessly day and night, William seems to be in a comparatively comfortable position brooding over her love for Scott. She seems to be quite less concerned when she discusses about the number of infant deaths in the camps. Even the children do not trust her as an individual. They agree to leave Scott and be with her, only when they consider her to be Scott's woman. Moreover, her behaviour towards the Indians is quite less compassionate than Scott who shows genuine love towards all. Kipling himself gave Scott the attributes of a demi-god when he writes, "a young man, beautiful as Paris, a god in a halo of golden dust, walking, slowly at the head of his flocks, while at his knee ran small naked Cupids." (Kipling 2015, 85).

Spivak has pointed out that the stories of Kipling which are based on tropical diseases, portray the image of the colonised as weak, invalid creatures at the mercy of the imperialists. His style of writing makes him unpopular among modern day readers. George Orwell denounces his work as "morally insensitive and aesthetically disgusting" (Rutherford 1964, 70), calling him a "jingo-imperialist" (Newsinger 1999, 11), while Spivak opposes his notions about the conquest of India to be a historically appropriate event. However, the stories of Kipling can be studied from a different perspective also. The stories are more of a direct account of the situations prevailing in British India than a reflection of his own thoughts and ideas. By portraying the attitudes and manners of the colonialists living in India, he also pointed out the several pretensions and superficiality of the imperialists.

Kipling cannot be considered as a bard of imperialism, rather, can be counted as a personality who explored and showed the British Empire in all its manifestations. Some of his poems like 'The White Man's Burden' can indeed be considered as reflecting a colonialist mentality and essentially a critique of colonialism. Instead of giving a judgement, he held out the situations to the readers and allowed them to draw their conclusions. It is for this reason that Kipling's works are subjected to varied interpretations. The works can be considered more as a social and colonial document, the retelling of incidents by a witness. Moreover,

William ultimately represents a figure of imperial power, the sovereign authority and her flaws bring out the flaws of an imperialist. Her interest in going back home for Christmas rather than staying to save lives brings out the true nature of a colonist. Moreover, with Faiz Ullah saving the life of his master, Scott, who almost falls a victim to the epidemic, the colonized too rises to the level of a saviour like his master. In sharp contrast to the character of Ram Dass in Kipling's short story 'By Word of Mouth', Faiz Ullah turns out to be an honest and faithful servant who never leaves his master alone. His Indian stories often bring out his views on Europe and India, as rightly summed up in 'The Ballad of East and West': " Oh, East is East, and West is West, and never the twain shall meet,/ Till Earth and Sky stand presently at God's great Judgement Seat;/ But there is neither East nor West, Border, nor Breed, nor Birth,/ When two strong men stand face to face, tho' they come from the ends of the earth!" (Kipling 2000, 26).

Kipling's short stories on tropical diseases can be rightly called, in the words of Priscilla Wald, "outbreak narratives" (Wald 2008, 2). She explains,

> The outbreak narrative- in its scientific, journalistic, and fictional incarnations- follows a formulaic plot that begins with the identification of an emerging infection, includes discussion of the global networks throughout which it travels, and chronicles the epidemiological work that ends with its containment.... Microbes, spaces, and interactions blend together as they animate the landscape and motivate the plot of the outbreak narrative: a contradictory compelling story of the perils of human interdependence and the triumph of human connection and cooperation, scientific authority and the evolutionary advantages of the microbe, ecological balance and impending disaster. (Wald 2008, 2)

Kipling's varied themes of paranormality, colonial masculinity etc. are constructed through a narrative of disease and contagion. Moreover, his detailed descriptions of the tropical diseases and the coloniser and colonised peoples' attitude towards them come from first-hand experience, although he had spent most of his life elsewhere. Though certain details provided in his stories are fictional, they do not fail to provide a concrete idea about diseases and healthcare.

The fumigatory powder used by Mellish in the story, *A Germ Destroyer* and the resultant thick black smoke might have been used solely for the sake of humour, but the idea cannot be rejected completely. The compound used to make the powder, that is, nitrate of strontia, indeed gives out thick black smoke as is seen while burning fire crackers that contain the compound. The entire idea of the fumigatory powder has been given a logical structure that adds on to the brilliance of the writer. Similarly, in the story, 'By Word of Mouth', we do not miss out on the logical explanations of death due to the outbreak of epidemics even though a paranormal theme has been inserted into it. Through a narrative of contagion, the story reflects the logical and fictional substances contained in it. Even in a controversial story like 'William the Conqueror', the medical problems that form the background of the story cannot be ignored. All the issues of patriarchy, colonialism, justifications and pretensions of imperialism can be understood in the light of the epidemic conditions. There can be no alternative reading of the texts where the issue of tropical diseases can be left out.

Kipling's works provide us with extensive materials to study healthcare and trace the developments of European medicine. Not only that, the implementation of the same and the gradual changes in the attitude towards them can also be understood from a clearer level. To study about European medicines and their usage in India, one has to begin with the diseases, their causes and effects. This can be best perceived in the works of Kipling. In 'Cholera Camp', he writes, "We've got to die somewhere—some way—some 'ow—/ We might as well begin to do it now!" (Kipling 1994, 456). Not only the diseases, but also the manner in which they are considered or accepted in a society comes out through his works. In his short story 'Love O'Women', the efforts of Tighe to conceal his 'disorder' considering the shame and social stigma attached to sexually transmitted diseases, bring out the psychological attitude towards certain illnesses. Again his own views towards illness has been brought out in *New Brooms*, "The wonder was not that men died like sheep, but that they did not die like flies; for their lives and their surroundings, their deaths, were part of a huge conspiracy against cleanliness" (Kipling 1909, 98).

Besides physical illness, mental illness too forms an important part of Kipling's writings. Many a time, he himself suffered from depression and was even on the verge of hanging himself. But it never stopped him from writing. Several stories and novels written by him bring out the depressions and suicidal tendencies of the characters. In *His Brother's Keeper*, one of the two men working in a canal attempts to commit suicide. The boy in 'Thrown Away', kills himself as he takes everything around him, too seriously. Even the character of Mowgli seems to be depressed in *The Spring Running* as he tries to run away from the unhappiness of his life. Kipling had also suffered from depression as a result of suffering from influenza for which he was advised to take a sea voyage. The depression felt by him and his family, while staying in the rented Rock House at Maidencombe near Torquay made him express it in *Something of Myself.* He also used this idea in *The House Surgeon*. But he could soon cope up with his depression and could give advices to others based on his experience. Several of his other works bring out the different aspects of mental illnesses alongwith the physical disorders.

To conclude, Kipling provides us with a wide array of fictional and non-fictional works based on diseases and healthcare. Though it can also be perceived in the works of other Victorian and early twentieth century writers like Philip Meadows Taylor and Flora Annie Steel,who is also called the "female Rudyard Kipling" (Mukherjee 2013, 95), it is in the works of Kipling that the fine threads of physical and mental illnesses are brought out. There is no doubt that the works of Kipling based on India are like a reservoir in which one has to delve deeper in order to understand the developments of a palliative, medically oriented imperialism.

REFERENCES

Beattie, James. 2011. *Empire and Environmental Anxiety: Health, Science, Art and Conservation in South Asia and Australasia, 1800-1920*. New York: Palgrave Macmillan.

Gillooly, Eileen. 2000. *Poetry for Young People: Rudyard Kipling*. New York: Sterling Publishing Company, Inc.

Kipling, Rudyard. 1884. *The Mark Of The Beast*. London: Orion Publishing Group.

Kipling, Rudyard. 1909. *Abaft The Funnel*. London: B.W. Dodge and Company.

Kipling, Rudyard. 1994. *The Collected Poems of Rudyard Kipling*. Hertfordshire: Wordsworth Editions Limited.

Kipling, Rudyard. 2015. *The Works of Rudyard Kipling*. London: Delphi Classics.

Kipling, Rudyard. 2016. *Plain Tales From The Hills*. London: Oxford University Press.

Kuokkanen, Rauna. 2007. *Reshaping The University: Responsibility, Indigenous Epistemes, and the Logic of the Gift*. Toronto: UBC Press.

Lancelyn Green, Roger. 1971. *Rudyard Kipling*. New York: Routledge.

Newsinger, John. 1999. *Orwell's Politics*. New York: Palgrave Macmillan.

Mukherjee, Upamanyu Pablo. 2013. *Natural Disasters and Victorian Empire: Famines, Fevers And The Literary Cultures Of South Asia*. New York: Palgrave Macmillan.

Pinney, Thomas. 1990. *The Letters of Rudyard Kipling*, Volume 2: 1890-99. New York: Palgrave Macmillan.

Rutherford, Andrew. 1964. Kipling's Mind and Art. Stanford (USA): Stanford University Press.

Wald, Priscilla. 2008. *Contagious Cultures, Carriers and the Outbreak Narrative*. Durham and London: Duke University Press.

In: Imperial Maladies
Editors: D. Bandyopadhyay et al.
ISBN: 978-1-53611-863-6

Chapter 6

BREAKING FREE OF THE DIALECTIC: AMITAV GHOSH'S *THE CALCUTTA CHROMOSOME* AS A CRITIQUE OF MODERNITY VIS-A-VIS COLONIAL MEDICAL SCIENCE

Pabitra Kumar Rana*
Department of English, Govt. General Degree College,
Dantan -II, Midnapore, West Bengal, India

I

Most of the novels of Amitav Ghosh are set against the backdrop of the British colonial occupation of India in the nineteenth and twentieth century. Having established their footmark in 1757 in Bengal and gradually overtaking the whole of India, the British ushered in a kind of

*Author's Address: Govt. General Degree College, Dantan -II, Midnapore, West Bengal, India. PIN: 721445. Email: rana.pabitra4@gmail.com.

Copernican Revolution in India. They became successful rulers in a vast and varied country like India not merely by force and violence but also by strategic introduction of modern institutions such as railway, law, public education, medicine etc. which have altered the Indian way of life. In other words, the British had introduced modernity in India. By modernity I mean the Western form of modernity which originated in post-medieval Europe. Though as a post-traditional order modernity can be understood in different ways in different disciplines ranging from Philosophy to Sociology and Aesthetics, as a historical category it refers to the post-Enlightenment period, characterised by rejection of tradition, rise of rationalism, technology, capitalism and individualism, development of the nation-state and its constituent institutions such as democracy, public education and bureaucracy and forms of surveillance. "In terms of history of philosophy," writes David Macey, "modernity is sometimes seen, as in Husserl, as being inaugurated by Descartes' vision of a philosophy and science that would make men the masters and possessors of nature (1637), but is usually made synonymous with the Enlightenment project and its belief that the light of reason and the natural sciences would eventually dispel the shadows and darkness of superstition, religion and political tyranny" (Macey 2000, 259-60). Central to the idea of modernity is the notion of the autonomy of the individual who would choose a course of action based on reason rather than on tradition. Interestingly, however, despite rationality being its operating principle, modernity has failed to replace the sureties of tradition by certitude of rational knowledge. Doubt is a pervasive component of modern critical reason, and permeates philosophical consciousness. "Modernity institutionalises," observes sociologist Anthony Giddens, "the principle of radical doubt and insists that all knowledge takes the form of hypotheses: claims which may very well be true, but which are in principle always open to revision and may have at some point to be abandoned" (Giddens 1991, 3). As a legacy of Enlightenment, modernity stands for, to quote Immanuel Kant, "the liberation of mankind from his self-caused state of minority." Apart from the emancipatory ethos enshrined in the notion of modernity, another very important but less recognized aspect of modernity is its role in colonial enterprise. Modernity's supposed potential to emancipate non-Europeans from primitivism has often been fielded as colonialism's justifiable logic of "civilising mission."

In *Colonial Modernity: Indian perspectives* (2011), the editor Pradip Basu describes colonial modernity as "the paradoxical reception of the European project of Enlightenment modernity by the rest of the world, whereby non-Europeans are assigned subject-ness precisely at the moment of the denial of their historical agency" (Basu 2011, 1). The role of science in establishing British colonialism in India in eighteenth and nineteenth centuries and in the birth of modern India was significant because science became not only technical authority but also cultural authority envisioning freedom and enlightenment, power and progress. Gyan Prakash observes that

> Standing as a metaphor for the triumph of universal reason over enchanting myths, science appears pivotal in the imagination and institution of India, a defining part of its history as a British colony and its emergence as an independent nation. (Prakash 1999, 3)

Western medicine can be viewed as a bedrock of British imperialism as it played a crucial role in confirming the supposed intellectual supremacy of the British over the Indians. The ushering of the institutions of colonial modernity at first impresses one as imperial altruism, but on deeper analysis they turn out to be tools of empire. In his influential book *Colonizing the Body* (1993), David Arnold observes that the highly prestigious Western medicine was one of the key players—others like penology, anthropology, the army, factory etc. being there—in the colonising process. For colonial medical science, body became a desired and contested site to achieve legitimacy. Arnold writes:

> Colonialism used or attempted to use the body as a site for the construction of its own authority, legitimacy and control. In part, therefore, the history of colonial medicine, and of the epidemic diseases with which it was so closely entwined, serves to illustrate the more general nature of colonial power and knowledge and to illuminate its hegemonic as well as its coercive process. Over the long period of British

> rule in India, the accumulation of medical knowledge about the body contributed to the political evolution and ideological articulation of the colonial system. Thus, medicine cannot be regarded as merely a matter of scientific interest. It cannot meaningfully be abstracted from the broader character of the colonial order. (Arnold 1993, 8)

Despite its hegemonic ambition, argues Arnold, Western medicine struggled hard to establish itself among Indian people, and "had failed to make the transition from state medicine to public health" (Arnold 1993, 3) throughout the entire British reign in India. The reasons for this unacceptability of Western Medicine by Indian masses may be that it was confined to the small enclave of the army and the Europeans, and more importantly, India had nourished the ancient medical systems of Ayurveda and Yunani, whose practitioners (the *kavirajas*, the *vaidyas* and the *hakims*) were easily available even in remote areas. The Indians' fascination for and hatred of Western medicine are at the heart of "the dialectics of power and knowledge in colonial India" (Arnold 1993, 7). Mark Harrison, another historian of medicine, notes in his 1994 book *Public Health in British India: Anglo-Indian Preventive medicine 1859-1914*, that "Medicine's role as a 'tool of empire' is probably the most familiar theme in the historiography of colonial medicine to date, and has its origins in the writings of colonial medical officers and imperial politicians" (Harrison 1994, 2). In the colonial enterprise, medicine became an instrument of social control in the colonies, providing means of knowing the indigenous population as well as of framing policies of public health. The British managed to rule the vast and varied India not merely through military control, but by developing, what Bernard Cohn has called "colonial forms of knowledge." "In coming to India," writes Cohn, "they unknowingly and unwittingly invaded and conquered not only a territory but an epistemological space as well." (Cohn 1996, 4) But the criteria used by the British to comprehend India were European, based on science, which they employed in the form of certain "investigative modalities" such as economics, ethnology, tropical medicine, cartography etc. But the irony is that while the colonisers believed that they had complete power over the

Indians, resistance came from within these modern institutions, and even resistance is prior to power in many instances. Amitav Ghosh's *The Calcutta Chromosome* (1995) which is subtitled "a novel of fevers, delirium and discovery," and has often been deemed as a medical thriller, plays with Western medicine, medical practitioner and epistemologies to problematise the power dynamics between the coloniser and the colonised.

In colonial encounters, modernity must be understood not merely as a legitimating agency of colonialism on the ground of spreading the light of civilisation and progress, but also, as Michael Hardt and Antonio Negri put it, a power relation of domination and resistance between the dominant and the subordinated. "There is no modernity without coloniality," claims Walter Mingolo, "because coloniality is constitutive of modernity."[1]Coloniality is constituted of the same hierarchy that is at modernity's heart. Neither Europe nor the colony is the sole location of modernity; rather, modernity lies in the power relation that straddles the two. The forces of resistance which they term as "antimodernity" in their 2009 book *Commonwealth* are not "outside modernity but rather entirely internal to it, that is within the power relation" (Hardt and Negri 2009, 67). The encounter between the coloniser and the colonised is never one-way traffic; in fact, both sides are changed in the relation involving "processes of mixture and mutual transformation that result from the struggle of domination and resistance" (Hardt and Negri 2009, 68).

The problem with traditional colonial historiography is that, claim Hardt and Negri, it does not only ignore the contribution of highly developed precolonial civilisations to the so-called modern civilisations (as in the case of the Nahua to the Spanish in Mexico or the Iroquois to the U.S. Constitution), but it also willfully denies resistances from the colonised. Ranajit Guha thinks that it is a conjuring trick of colonial historiography "to make resistance disappear from political history of India under British rule."[2] This deliberate erasure of resistance comes close to

[1]Walter Mingolo, *The Idea of Latin America* (Cambridge: Blackwell, 2005), p.xiii. qtd. in *Comonwealth* by Michael Hardt and Antonio Negri, pp.67.

[2]RanajitGuha, *Dominion without Hegemony: History and Power in Colonial India* (Cambridge, Mass.: Harvard University Press, 1997), pp.89 qtd. in *Comonwealth* by Michael Hardt and Antonio Negri, pp.70.

the psychoanalytic idea of "foreclosure" by which the unpalatable histories are not admitted at all. Foreclosure differs from repression in that whereas the repressed element is forced inside the psyche where they remain buried deep, the foreclosed is expelled outside, so that the ego can function without any kind of inhibition, as if the incidents have not occurred at all. The denial by historiography of resistance from non-European peoples is a strategy to foreground the idea that modernity is a purely European invention. But ironically, resistances do not come from outside, but from inside. Hardt and Negri posit:

> The foreclosed element in this case is not only the history of contributions to modern culture and society by non-European peoples and civilizations, making it seem that Europe is the source of all modern innovation, but also and more important the innumerable *resistances* within and against modernity, which constitute the primary element of danger for its dominant self-conception. Despite all the furious energy expended to cast out the "antimodern" other, resistances remain within. (Hardt and Negri 2009, 70)

In order to comprehend how the resisting forces of antimodernity inhere within modernity, Hardt and Negri postulated three parameters. First, antimodernity is not an effort to glorify or preserve the premodern but a struggle for freedom within modernity. Second, "antimodernity is not external to but rather coextensive with modernity" (Hardt and Negri 2009, 101). The geographical centre-periphery model which constructs Europe as modern and colonies as antimodern fails when European history is found smeared with various slave rebellions, peasant protests, proletarian resistances and other movements, and at the same time, highly developed and complex forms of social organisations are discovered in colonial world. Third, in terms of temporality, antimodernity does not come after modernity, as a reaction to modernity's hegemonic power; rather, "antimodernity is prior in the sense that the power relation of modernity can be exercised only over free subjects who express that freedom through resistance to hierarchy and domination"(Hardt and Negri 2009, 101).Their understanding of modernity as power relation also undermines Jurgen

Habermas' notion of modernity as an unfinished project because completing the unfinished project of modernity would only produce the structure of domination and subordination. Rather, resistances which they term as "antimodernity" are internal to modern domination.

As examples of foreclosure for modernity's self-conception, Hardt and Negri refer to the strategy of the modern republic of property to make the presence of slavery and racism—despite these two being the cornerstones of the republic's economy and chauvinistic optimism—disappear from its history, or, if acknowledged at all, to dismiss them as mere aberrations to the republic's core ideological principles of equality and freedom. So modernity is as much constituted by coloniality as by racism; the three—modernity, coloniality and racism—form a complex, the modernity-coloniality-racism triumvirate whose techniques and instruments permeate subordinated populations not merely in the abstract ideological level but also in practical, day to day practices of life. As for the all-pervasive impact of the modernity-coloniality-racism complex, reference may be made to Edward Said's influential study of Orientalism which demonstrates how the representations of the colonised in novels, histories, administrative documents and a host of other texts not only legitimise colonial rule but also mould the very consciousness of the colonised as inferior. Gayatri Spivak also provocatively claims that in the hegemonic structure of colonialism and patriarchy, the subaltern cannot speak whose voice is either ideologically silenced or appropriated by the dominant class. Colonialism accomplished, it seems, its task of complete domination not merely through violence, but more effectively through tacit consent from the colonised by making them internalise colonial forms of knowledge and values. But despite the all-pervasive colonial biopower which invests both the forms of consciousness and forms of life of the dominated peoples, it fails to occlude resistances from them. External forms of resistances such as violent revolt could reverse the hierarchy of the coloniser and the colonised; but resistances could be more subtle and nuanced when it is prior to power. Amitav Ghosh's science-fiction *The Calcutta Chromosome* (1996) is a nuanced commentary on the power relation between the coloniser and the colonised; it is a power relation in which the supposed power of modernity and colonialism fails to contain the natives who seem to embody resistances of antimodernity prior to colonial subjection. The article aims to understand how the natives not only dismantle the hierarchical power relation of modernity and antimodernity but also break free—very ingeniously, without staging any kind of crude external resistances—of the entire dialectic of modernity and antimodernity, and envisions, what Hardt and Negri term "altermodernity," through forming alternative medical system and embracing forms of subjectivities which defy the Western notion of rational self and identity.

II

Set in the uncertain future of early twenty first century, in *The Calcutta Chromosome* Ghosh traces—via Ava, the super computer of Antar, a New York based employee of International Water Council—the mystery of L. Murugan, a former colleague of Antar at Lifewatch and a diehard malaria enthusiast who disappeared at Calcutta on 21 August in 1995. Antar's stumbling upon an old ID card of L.Murugan on Ava's screen leads him to excavate—through futuristic cybernetic surveillance and reminiscences involving complex network of events spanning across centuries and continents—an alternative history of the British medical doctor Ronald Ross' discovery of malaria parasite at Calcutta in 1898. Ross was awarded the Nobel Prize in 1902 for his breakthrough in malaria research, and since then has been hailed as a great scientist. As per the official version, Ross was a rare genius who undertook the research to save humanity from the world's oldest and probably the most widespread disease, malaria. But Murugan shows Ross was neither a genius nor was his work motivated by any humanitarian urge. Ross was, opined Murugan in a mockingly irreverent tone to Antar, both a genius and a dickhead, the least likely person to discover anything, let alone malaria parasite. Murugan constructs his narrative by building on Ross's biography and his memoir as well as from a host of other sources, mainly letters and e-mails of different persons involved in the story. He states young Ross aspired to be a poet, and also liked enjoying the youth and the world; he was a "Colonial type" (47) who loved hunting, playing tennis and polo, grew thick moustache on his chubby pink cheeks, drank whisky for breakfast. Ghosh's portrayal of Ross corresponds to that of Mark Harrison who writes that as a young recruit Ross had "little predilection for medicine," and he joined the Indian Medical Service because "his father (an Indian Army General) had urged him to do so, and because it afforded excellent sporting opportunities – especially fishing, polo, and pig-sticking" (13-14). As the official version has it, after two years of joining the Indian Medical Service, one fine morning Ross decided that he would solve the malaria mystery, and jumped into his research in which he achieved breakthrough in three years. But Murugan discredits the official narrative, and claims that Ross was motivated to undertake the malaria research as a colonial project by Dr. Patrick Manson, the discoverer of filarial parasite and who was the Queen's head honcho in bacteriology. He knew that malaria was the research priority of the day and the research on it was important in the competition among European countries in colonial expansion. By building on the progress made by Alphonse Laveran, Dr. Manson believed that malaria was transmitted from mosquito dust via drinking water. He sent Ross to India to do the research in order to "carry the torch for the Queen and the Empire" (61). But the most significant part of Murugan's research is his hypothesis that "some other person or persons had systematically interfered with Ronald Ross's experiments to push malaria research in certain directions while leading it away from others" (32-3). According to Murugan, Ross was manipulated by a secret group of natives in making the malaria breakthrough by guiding him in particular direction. When Ross was almost hopeless about getting samples of malaria blood in Begumpett near Secunderabad, a man called Abdul Kadir dropped by to volunteer, and then a guy named Lutchman came in who became the de facto supervisor of Ross. It is this Lutchman who not only disproved Dr. Manson's hypothesis but also casually pointed out to Ross that malaria is caused by a particular species of mosquito, anopheles. Murugan believes that Abdul Kadir and Lutchman are members of a secret group of low-caste natives headed by a woman named Mangala. The crux of Murugan's narrative is that this group was streets ahead in malaria research than Ross, and that they had their unique knowledge-system which functioned on the principle that to know something is to change it. Murugan guessed that they were struck in some point of their secret research and the only way they can move to the next step was through a mutation in malaria parasite which can only be achieved through making the previous developments public. Mangala's discovery that malaria parasite carries the randomly assorted personality traits of the infected person via pigeon into another person's body is the crucial knowledge that helps her to achieve the ultimate thing, the transcendence of nature, that is, immortality. Murugan observes that the two persons—the linguist J.W.D. Grigson and the young bacteriologist Elijah Farley—who almost discovered the secret workings of Lutchman and Mangala are scared away and murdered. Even D.D. Cunnigham, who employed Mangala, disappeared mysteriously from Calcutta. Ross suited them because he was absolutely oblivious of what was happening around him; he never enquired who the natives really were or where are they from. To him, they were mere servants, ignorant people who do not deserve attention from a scientist like him. Even just when Luthcman told him that malaria vector might be one species of mosquito which he never imagined, his immediate response was one of sahib-like reprimanding of the natives: "next time I want your help I'll ask for it"(68). After making the discovery, Ross thanks Angel of Fate rather than suspecting Lutchman and enquiring how an uneducated fellow like him got to know this crucial idea. He naively believed Lutchman when the latter passes it as to have learnt from some villagers up the Nilgiri hills. Murugan relishes the irony as do the readers: "He thinks he's doing experiments on the malaria parasite. And all the time it's he who *is* the experiment on the malaria parasite" (69). Ross imbued racial notion of European supremacy so much that he did not bother about his assistant at all; he believed that the British were "superior to subject peoples in natural ability, integrity and science…They [had] introduced honesty, law, justice, order, roads, posts, railways, irrigation, hospitals…and what was necessary for civilization, a final superior authority" (Memoirs, 17; qtd. in Harrison). The novel upsets the apple cart for a racist-imperialist like Ross who is exposed as a dolt and mere tool in the hands of a group of natives.

That Ghosh has challenged the Western cultural hegemony and deconstructed the binary of superiority and inferiority between the West and East have been pointed out by some critics. Claire Chambers views the novel as a postcolonial science fiction which undermines the universalist claim of Western science by mixing fact with fiction, and by fictionally showing how Ross was manipulated by a counter-scientific Indian group which was much advanced in malaria research. Chambers also argues that Ross' discovery was as much predicated upon reason as on faith. In her analysis "the novel seems to suggest that all forms of scientific knowledge are in fact provisional, they are stories being told, still mutating like the malaria parasite" (Chambers 2003, 69). Isabella Bruschi has argued that Ghosh has deconstructed the dichotomy between official Western science and alternative Eastern science but has avoided the risk of revised essentialism by making the narrator partly reliable. The novel endorses, according to her, the view that "a fusion between official and alternative forms of knowledge can be a way out of the opposing and excluding constraints of colonial discourse" (Bruschi 2009, 78). John Thieme rejects both the post-colonial critics' Manichean views regarding colonial discourse and the hybridization model proposed by Bhabha as both of these tend to forget the local specifics, and instead contends that Ghosh is concerned to excavate a labyrinthine network of traces, which foreground such specifics, while making it clear that essentialist versions of national and regional cultures, such as those inherent in Orientalist discourses, are unsustainable. Ghosh's purpose in this fiction is to open up a discursive and imaginative space for giving voice to hitherto silenced subalterns. "Throughout the text," observes Thieme, "readers are made aware that the borderline between discoverers and those who are discovered is an extremely porous one" (Thieme 2003, 139) as are evident in the cases of Ross and Mangala, Murugan and Antar, Murugan and Urmila, and finally, Antar and the readers. The ultimate discoverer who is discovered by the novel is the reader who has to piece together the text's numerous clues to arrive at least at one of the possible versions of meaning. Tabish Khair examines the question of subaltern agency in the narrative by locating the Indian English writer in the privileged, upper caste Babu class while most of the Indians belong to the illiterate, underprivileged Coolie class. Khair rightly recognizes the problem—in the vein of Gayatri Spivak— of the writer/narrator who will narrate the agency of the subaltern subjects who belong to the discourse outside the discourse which constitutes the writer/narrator. Ghosh has achieved a remarkable feat, according to Khair, by raising the issue of subaltern agency without appropriating their voice. For this Ghosh avoids the vulgar dualism of Science and Magic, Man and Machine in order to show the shadow lines that construct these binaries. The secret procedure of Mangala' group cannot be discarded as irrational though it is incomprehensible to the Western rationality. The "other" versions of ir/rationality are epitomized, argues Khair, in the human sacrifice which is construed by the European rationality as the extreme sign of barbarity and irrationality of non-European cultures. But in the novel, human sacrifice is generative of new bodies, new identities. The inability of Cunningham and Ross to comprehend the agency of the subaltern group is failure of colonial rationality in "alien" space which is called India. The power of the coloniser and powerlessness of the natives are exposed as fiction. "Ghosh," writes Khair, "clearly recognises that power (in political and economic senses) remains the prerogative of the coloniser, but he also explores through fiction the ways in which the colonised, the subaltern can subvert this power" (Khair 2003, 156).In the second chapter entitled "The 'metaphysic' of modernity" of his monograph *Amitav Ghosh*(2010) Anshuman A. Mondal focuses on Ghosh's take on modernity in general and in *The Circle of Reason, In An Antique Land* and *The Calcutta Chromosome* in particular. Mondal reads Ghosh's novels as to how they negotiate the Western knowledge as a contested site. Mondal deems *The Calcutta Chromosome* as Ghosh's strategy to reverse the authority of colonial science to challenge the diffusionist "narrative of scientific discovery whereby knowledge travels out from the Western centre to the non-Western periphery" (Mondal 2010, 54). He identifies three displacements whereby the reversal is accomplished. First, instead of any first world city, Calcutta, a colonial city from a third-world country is the site of scientific research. Second, the scientific authority is shifted from the colonial scientists to the subaltern group. Third, there is a dismantling of the Western form of knowledge which claims to be the only legitimate form of epistemology. And lastly, Mondal focuses on the paradox of the "impossible" native knowledge which eludes recognition. While such readings highlight Ghosh's critique of colonial discourse by reversing and dismantling it without endorsing reversed essentialism, they do not take into account the novel's potential to undermine the self-certified universality and legitimacy of colonial modernity through fictionally empowering the natives who not merely manifest antimodern resistances by virtue of their preexisting freedom but also break free of the oppositional stance of modernity and antimodernity and move—along a diagonal line that escapes the confining play of opposites—from resistance to alternative.

III

Going by Murugan's claims, the subaltern group's quest for immortality is predicated upon interpersonal transference: the disposition of a malaria-infected person is transmitted to a recipient when the blood of the donor is injected in the syphilis-hit recipient's body. In fact, using malaria parasite was the standard procedure for syphilis treatment in the West for long before the advent of penicillin; and though discovering this procedure of treating disease with disease fetched Julius von Wagner-Jauregg the Nobel in 1927, he did not know, claims Murugan, how it actually worked in human body. Coincidentally, Mangala used the same procedure of injecting malarial blood to cure syphilitic paresis but with a twist: she used pigeons—like test-tube or agar plate—for "making the bug cross over" before injecting the malarial blood in syphilis-hit patient. She discovered personality transpositions in this procedure which worked because of asexual transfer of what Murugan calls the Calcutta chromosome which affects the brain only. In this way, a person can continue to exist in newer incarnations through chromosome transfer in the "chosen." Interestingly, the recipient can comprehend the entire process after the transposition is achieved. Thus, the mechanism remains ever secret. What is at stake in Mangala's system is the ontology of the persons involved. The novel endorses the kind of selfhood which is multiple, fragmentary, and always is in the process of evolution. The process of migratory selfhood is elaborated by Murugan:

> '...when your body fails you, you leave it, you migrate—you or at least a matching symptomology of your self. You begin all over again, another body...'(95)

Chitra Sankaran notes that in the novel the sameness of the self is left "un-circumscribed" and "fluid". This un-circumscribed self also defies the constraints of time and space.

The kind of autonomous selfhood and mode of existence embodied in the secret group's lived experience come close to Hardt and Negri's notion of "altermodernity" which is marked by a decisive break with modernity and its hierarchical power relation as well as extending beyond the opposition and resistance of antimodernity. Altermodernity is truly revolutionary in the sense that it rejects both modernity's domination and antimodernity's oppositional affirmation of identity and tradition; thus, discrediting any sort of fixed identity, altermodernity favours "becoming" over static "being." Whereas the passage from modernity to antimodernity leads to static stance of opposition, the passage from antimodernity to altermodernity is characterised by transformation involving "rupture with any fixed dialectic between modern sovereignty and antimodern resistance" (Hardt and Negri 2009, 106). That is why Claire Chambers' contention that "Ghosh projects the possibility of the Hindu doctrine of reincarnation becoming a material reality in the future"(Chambers 2003, 59) seems untenable because such a stance—despite its focus on unstuck selfhood— aligns Ghosh with antimodernity; rather, "the most important point in *The Calcutta Chromosome* is that," writes Suparno Banerjee, "in bringing together the scientific and the spiritual elements, and also in subverting Western epistemology, it does not employ classical Hindu mythology or invoke traditional Vedic knowledge"(Banerjee 2010, 58). Similarly, the novel discredits the Western medicine and exposes the intellectual inferiority of its practitioners but without falling back and glorifying the traditional Indian medicine of Ayurveda and Yunani. Syphilis patients visit PG Hospital not to meet Cunningham or Ross but to see Mangala who treats them under the nose of noted colonial doctors. Mangala's method of treatment is neither entirely Western nor Indian system of medicine; she appropriates Western microscopy but practices it in conjunction with mysticism. The syphilis patients who came to her at the backyard of Cunningham's laboratory chant—by squatting around a fire— in unison "to the accompaniment of hand-held brass cymbals, as though in preparation for a ritual or ceremony" (129). Mangala sat alone on a low divan at the far end of the room in an attitude of command, and beside her were many bamboo cages containing a pigeon each. Elijah Farley who found out the mysterious activities of Mangala could not bring him to believe that a sweeper woman can treat syphilis and be worshipped by the patients; he dubs her as "a false prophetess" (130) who cheated sick, poor people of money they could ill afford. What is more, both Mangala and Lutchman belong to the lowest stratum of Indian society; Lutchman is a low-caste whom the upper-caste station master tried to kill, and Mangala is a sweeper woman. As for Mangala, who is the chief brain of the native group, she is never looked upon seriously; she is taken for granted as a figure of third-world woman who disappears between patriarchy and imperialism. Even modernity's emphasis on autonomy of subjects takes only men as free subjects, excluding women from subjectivity. Kanchana Mahadevan thinks that in the context of Indian colonialism the British thinkers like J.S. Mill and James Mill considered Indian society as barbaric which was "especially testified in the inferior condition of Indian women taking to sati and the alleged effeminacy of Indian men"(199). Interestingly, though the rise of nationalism propagated the need for strong women by invoking the image of superwomen (a combination of the spiritual Maitreyi, the learned Gargi, the suffering Sita, the faithful Savitri and the heroic Lakshmibai), it was constructed on the image of high caste women, excluding the lower-caste. Kanchana Mahadevan puts it succinctly:

> Yet as this superwoman fought for her nation, her own others, namely, the washerwomen, the domestic servants, the wet-nurses, the lower caste, the Muslim and Christian women were forgotten – in short, the 'vedic dasi' was overlooked in the homogenization of Indian women in the project of modern nationalism. (Mahadevan 2002, 201)

A woman like Mangala figures nowhere – be it in the imaginative boundary of the coloniser or of the colonised. Murugan identifies them as "fringe people, marginal types" who are so far from the mainstream that one cannot "see them from the shore" (92).They were already marginalized within the caste-obsessed Indian society. But they knew all about Ross and a lot about the best collection of parasites. They turned their invisibility in Indian society and in high-browed colonial ideology into an opportunity to continue their research unrecognised and uninterrupted. By covertly building their own form of medicine and modernity, they resist and move beyond the hegemonic structures (such as science/superstition, mainstream/marginal, central/peripheral etc.) endorsed by both Indian society and colonial discourse.

By virtue of their knowledge system which functions without articulation, the members of the secret cult reincarnate themselves in newer identities across the collapse of time and space. As for the identity of Lutchman, Murugan clarifies to Antar: "'Too many may be. As I see it, he was all over the map, changing names, switching identities'"(76). Lutchman who appears at Ross' laboratory in Begumpett in 1895 and remains his servant for the next three years may be linked to Laakhan who – as Phulboni came to know while passing a macabre night at Renupur station in 1933 – used to stay at Renupur station, and who arranged for the murder of the station master in 1860s, and who is the probable murderer of Elijah Farley in 1894. It is the same Laakhan whose reincarnations are Romen Halder of Kolkata in 1995 and Lucky of New York in indefinite future. Similarly, the Armenian Mrs. Aratounian who lives in Calcutta, the hard-working and self-dependent Calcutta journalist Urmila Roy and the New York babysitter Tara in future are all avatars of Mangala across temporal and spatial barriers. These characters occupy different identities in different times and different places but with some basic trait (Lutchman's missing thumb, for example) linking all incarnations. Mangala is at the same time a sweeper woman and a goddess among her devotees; she is worshipped long after she migrates from her original body as the little girl of Kalighat innocently passes the secret: "Today is the last day of the puja of Mangala–bibi. Baba says that tonight Mangala-bibi is going to enter a new body" (200). Murugan thinks that her syphilis-infected patients cum devotees might have believed her to be "a witch or a magician or a god or whatever" (210). Similarly Lutchman is apparently a servant of the British Government, a dhooley-bearer whose job was to shovel shit, and he acted as an obedient personal servant of Ross. But all his jobs are nothing but role-playing of the inscrutable front-man of Mangala'a cult. He is ever enigmatic, right from his boyhood at Renupur station to his association with Ross to the ingratiating Lucky. The uniqueness of the natives is that their subjectivity is integrally related, and in a sense, is the effect of their own knowledge system which may be discredited and disqualified by the dominant knowledge system but which, nonetheless, is efficacious in empowering the natives. This indigenous knowledge system chimes with what Michel Foucault has called—in the first (delivered on 7 January, 1976) of his "Two Lectures"—"the insurrection of subjugated knowledges." By "subjugated knowledges," Foucault refers to

> a whole set of knowledges that that have been disqualified as inadequate to their task or insufficiently elaborated: naïve knowledges, located low down on the hierarchy, beneath the required level of cognition or scientificity. (Foucault 1980, 82)

Foucault thinks that criticism performs its task through the reemergence of the disqualified knowledge. The novel itself performs the task of critiquing colonial medical science by staging a hypothetical reemergence of indigenous knowledge system which should not be confused with any ancient or premodern knowledge system of India. Rather, Mangala develops her system by drawing both from Western microscopy and Indian mystical tradition. As a researcher, Murugan's findings can be seen as genealogy which from Foucauldian perspective can be described as, writes Clare O' Farrell, "a form of research aimed at activating 'subjugated' historical knowledge, that is, knowledge which has been rejected by mainstream knowledge, or which is too local or specific to be deemed of any importance" (68). The function of genealogy is to pay attention to "local, discontinuous, disqualified, illegitimate knowledges against the unitary body of theory" (83), and to reactivate them into play. Foucault cautions us that genealogy is not against the "contents, methods or concepts of a science" but against the homogenizing, centralising power of scientific discourse. Mangala's method which Murugan disinters and which he dubs as "anti-science" is not accredited by the Western science but is none the less effective in not merely curing syphilis but in interpersonal transference across spatial-temporal collapse. But once excavated, does not the knowledge system of the secret group run the risk of being appropriated and re-codified by the dominant discourse or being placed in dialectical opposition against the dominant discourse? If such were the case, then genealogies are likely to be hoisted in their own petard. Foucault chalks out the tentative mechanism of genealogies:

> At all events, we must proceed just as if we had not alarmed them at all, in which case it will be no part of our concern to provide a solid and homogenous theoretical terrain for all these dispersed genealogies, nor to descend upon them from on high with some kind of halo of theory that would unite them. Our task, on the contrary, will be *to expose and specify the issue at stake in this opposition, this struggle, this insurrection of knowledges against the institutions and against effects of the knowledge and power that invests the scientific discourse.* (Foucault 1980, 87) [emphases mine]

This is what Mangala's system does; she never attempts to reverse the hierarchy. Instead, she runs her system in such a way that it remains beyond the cognition of the colonisers who are left to wallow in their cosy illusion. Here, once again, the power of the natives precedes that of the coloniser, and in a sense, eludes the dialectical trap of modernity and primitivism. Though Murugan tries to clarify the workings of the secret group on the basis of the oppositional model of "Christ and anti-Christ," "science and counter-science," (91) the novel proposes an alternative beyond the opposition between science and anti-science, between modernity and antimodernity. From the narrative perspective, the novel does not make any authentic claim as the alternative narrative is predicated upon the hypothesis of an unreliable narrator who, though claims to be an authority on the medical history of malaria, has only "one of the ways of putting it,"(51) and repeatedly admits his struggle to see the whole truth. Murugan tries to establish connections among events spanning across centuries and continents, and he constructs his narrative based on a series of hypothetical propositions as are evident from his hesitations[" 'The truth is,' he said, 'that I don't know..." (184); "We don't even know what we don't know" (185); "I am just guessing wildly here. Okay?"(211); "'My hunch is that she found some way of making the bird cross over, so that the bird could be used like a test-tube, or an agar plate"(212) and "All I have is bits and pieces—no beginning, no middle and definitely no end"(215)] while narrating his version to Antar and Urmila. The rejection of his paper "An Alternative Interpretation of Late 19th Century Malaria Research: is there a Secret History?" by the scientific community and the revocation of his membership from the History of Science Society are indications of how the alternate versions are discredited till now, but which continue to exist in palimpsest.

From the Postcolonial point of view, one cannot miss the irony: colonial scientists think the natives to be ever obeying, faithful and ignorant subjects upon whom they can test their hypothesis, whom they can employ as servants, upon whom they have complete control, and whom they did not think important enough to mention in their diaries and memoirs; but they turn out to be much clever, intelligent people who are out of the loop of the hegemony of modernity and colonialism. In a sense, these fringe people form an alterity, an unassimilable other that both resists and breaks free of modernity's notion of self and identity. To the coloniser, the colonies may be like laboratories of modernity in which the colonisers were scientists and the colonised the mice and guinea pigs. But interestingly, these laboratories may also be, as Diane M. Nelson observes, sites of slippage where each "element may act in multifarious ways, modifying, appropriating, ignoring, mutating" (254).

If modernity is not only ideological, but also material, practical forms of life, then the subaltern group lives up to it from the reverse side. Mangala and her followers not only devise the mechanism of fluid selfhood which defies modernity's notion of time and space but also live, experience, experiment and exist in it. In the migratory process, body is the primary locus for reincarnations, and in a sense, their bodies escape the grip of the colonisers. Their bodies no longer remain, as Arnold called, contested site, and become autonomous terrain. The passage from anti- to altermodernity is both epistemological and ontological. The trajectory of altermodernity extends towards—by continual rupture with past—a new future "where Becoming is prior to Being," and where identity is a constant process of "becoming other" (124). The secret group's ever-evolving epistemology (to be at par with the changing nature of malaria parasite) and the migratory, liminal selfhood Mangala and members of her secret cult live through come close, ironically perhaps, to Giddens' proposition that the knowledge of modernity is always open to revision. But the modernity the native group envisions is alternative form of modernity, not what Giddens thought it to be.

References

Arnold, David. 1993. *Colonizing the Body: State Medicine and Epidemic Disease in Nineteenth-century India*. Berkeley: University of California Press.

Banerjee, Suporno. 2010. "The Calcutta Chromosome: A Novel of silence, Slippage and Subversion." In *Science Fiction, Imperialism and the Third World: Essays on Postcolonial Literature and Film*, edited by

Erica Hoagland and Reema Sarwal. 50-64. Jefferson: McFarland & Company.

Basu, Pradip, ed. 2011. *Colonial Modernity: Indian perspectives*. Kolkata: Setu Prakashini.

Bruschi, Isabella. 2009. "The Calcutta Chromosome: Reading Western Cultural Hegemony." In *Amitav Ghosh: Critical Essays*, edited by Bibhash Choudhury. 65-80. New Delhi: PHI

Chambers, Claire. 2003. "Postcolonial Science Fiction: Amitav Ghosh's The Calcutta Chromosome." *Journal of Commonwealth Literature*, 57-72. Accessed January 17, 2017.jcl.sagepub.com/../58.full.pdf

Cohn, Bernard S. 1996. *Colonialism and its Forms of Knowledge*. Princeton: Princeton University Press.

Foucault, Michel. 1980. "Two Lectures" in *Power/Knowledge: Selected Interviews and Other Writings, 1972-1977*, edited by Colin Gordon. Trans. Colin Gordon, Leo Marshall, John Mepham, Kate Soper. 78-92. New York: Pantheon Books.

Ghosh, Amitav. 1996. *The Calcutta Chromosome*. New Delhi: Penguin.

Giddens, Anthony. 1991. *Modernity and Self-Identity*. Stanford (USA): Stanford University Press.

Hardt, Michael and Antonio Negri. 2009. *Commonwealth*. Massachusetts (USA): Harvard University Press.

Harrison, Mark. 1994. *Public Health in British India: Anglo-Indian Preventive Medicine 1859-1914*. Cambridge: Cambridge University Press.

Khair, Tabish. 2003. "Amitav Ghosh's The Calcutta Chromosome: The Question of Subaltern Agency." In *Amitav Ghosh: A Critical Companion,* edited by Tabish Khair. 142-161. Delhi: Permanent Black.

Khair, Tabish. 2003. *Amitav Ghosh: A Critical Companion*, edited by Tabish Khair. 128-141. Delhi: Permanent Black.

Macey, David. 2000. *The Penguin Dictionary of Critical Theory*. London: Penguin.

Mahadevan, Kanchana. 2002. "Colonial Modernity: A Critique," *IndianLiterature,* 46. 3 (209), (May-June, 2002), 193-211. Accessed May 16, 2016. www.jstor.org/stable/29998618.

Mondal, Anshuman A. 2010. *Amitav Ghosh*. Manchester (UK): Manchester University Press.

Nelson, Diane M. 2003. "A Social Science Fiction of Fevers, Delirium and Discovery: The Calcutta Chromosome, the Colonial Laboratory, and the Postcolonial New Human," *Science Fiction Studies*, 30.2, Social Science Fiction, 245-266. Accessed December 29, 2016. www.jstor.org/stable/4241117.

O'Farrell, Clare. 2005. *Michel Foucault*. London: Sage.

Prakash, Gyan. 1999. *Another Reason: Science and the Imagination of Modern India*. Princeton: Princeton University Press.

Sankaran, Chitra. 2012. "Sharing Landscapes and Mindscapes: Ethics and Aesthetics in Amitav Ghosh's The Calcutta Chromosome." In History, *Narrative and Testimony in Amitavghosh's Fiction*, edited by ChitraSankaran. 109-119.Albany: State University of New York Press

Thieme, John. 2003. "The Discover Discovered: Amitav Ghosh's The Calcutta Chromosome." In *Amitav Ghosh: A Critical Companion,* edited by TabishKhair. 128-141. Delhi: Permanent Black.

In: Imperial Maladies
Editors: D. Bandyopadhyay et al.
ISBN: 978-1-53611-863-6

Chapter 7

TROPICAL DISEASES AND HELPLESS COLONIAL RESPONSES: MEDICAL HUMANISM IN GREENE'S *JOURNEY WITHOUT MAPS* AND FARRELL'S *THE SIEGE OF KRISHNAPUR*

Ujjwal Kr. Panda*
Dept. of English, Govt. General Degree College, Dantan-II,
Paschim Medinipur, West Bengal, India

Medical Humanism is a relatively new development that achieved currency in North America towards the beginning of this century and attempts an understanding of medicines beyond the well-known stereotype of medicine as a care-based and evidence-based discipline. It explores the social, cultural and historical dimensions of medicines and seeks to represent medicines predominantly as a value-based field. At the very least, it provides an interdisciplinary, as well as an interprofessional,

*Author's Address: Govt. General Degree College, Dantan –II, Kashmuli, Paschim Medinipur, West Bengal, India. PIN 721445. Email: biju.ujjwal@gmail.com.

attempt to examine and understand the unmistakable effects of ailments and disease on patients, health professionals and the society itself into which they live and work. It also includes humanities like literature, philosophy, history, religion and ethics and social sciences such as anthropology, cultural studies, sociology, health geography and psychology to show the development of the application of medical theories in them and to record how the immensity of diseases and medical endeavours to avert them form a substantial part in their evolution. Medical Humanism is marked by an intense love for human beings which is more intent on considering disease as a suffering rather than being a set of symptoms. It tries to focus upon the psychology of the patients and the medical professionals to show that diseases tend to exist on a humanistic level beyond the fundamentally bio-scientific model of human medicines. In recent times, the need for an integration of humanistic and scientific spirits of medicines is gradually realized. Fuquing Gong, Yupeng Diao, Taowen Pan, Min Liu and Hongliang Sun emphasize this need in their essay, "Evolution of Human Medical Model and Development Course of Medical Humanistic Spirit" -

> During medical practice, medical humanistic spirit and medical scientific spirit should be integrated, complementary and mutually reinforcing. Medical science alleviates and heals patients' diseases, while medical humanistic spirit provides psychological support to patients. Medical science can only deal with physical suffering of patients through advanced technological means, while medical humanistic spirit can appease patients' psychological trauma. Humans are composed of mind and body; in order to fully and completely resolve the suffering of patients, the two must supplement and complement each other. (Gong et al. 2015, 413)

But what happens when a particular geographical territory is marked by a total absence or an utter collapse of "advanced technological means" of medical science? In the present chapter I would like to show that peculiar condition when Medical Humanistic spirit becomes the only saving spirit in the face of immense severity of disease and human suffering in relation to Graham Greene's 1936- travelogue, *Journey without Maps* and J. G. Farrell's novel, *The Siege of Krishnapur* (1973). Of course the texts deal with different geographies and diseases and their modes of representing medical humanism are fundamentally different from each other. At the same time one can refer to the basic difference between the representation of actual reality of the West African Republic of Liberia in *Journey without Maps* and the fictional reality of an imaginary North Indian town, Krishnapur, during the Indian Mutiny of 1857 in Farrell's novel. But both the works are deeply embedded into the ground reality of two continents of two different times. *The Siege of Krishnapur* is a beautiful example of historical metafiction because it fictionalises the sieges of Cawnpore (now Kanpur) and Lucknow where a besieged British garrison succeeds in resisting the attack of the native sepoys for about four months amidst inhuman suffering before being finally relieved. In his Afterword of the novel Farrell has admitted his metafictive leanings when he confesses his debt to the historians of Indian Mutiny like Maria Germon, Rev. H. S. Polehampton, F. C. Scherer, Mark Thornhill and others. So the two books in a way show the inability of the imperial and bio-scientific medical models to cure tropical diseases and referring to the psychology of the patients open up the possibility of an intersection of medicine and literature.

"The motive of a journey deserves a little attention. It is not the fully conscious mind which chooses West Africa in preference to Switzerland" (Greene 1980, 20), writes Graham Greene towards the beginning of *Journey without Maps* which records his a 350-mile and almost one-month-long walk through the interiors of the West African Republic of Liberia in 1935 along with his cousin Barbara and a large group of native carriers. The typical imperial apprehension about Africa, a largely uncharted territory by then (resultantly marked by a fear of the unknown), reminds us of the remarks of the old doctor at Brussels who asks Marlow, the hero of Conrad's *Heart of Darkness,* in an amusing but matter-of-fact tone- "Ever any madness in your family?" after coming to know about his intention to go to the Congo Basin. *Heart of Darkness* has been a focal point in Greene's book and there are recurring references to the so called heart of darkness in it. Surely, Greene went there on a spy mission on behalf of the British Anti-Slavery Movement to investigate allegations that Liberia, a state born as a refuge for freed American slaves, was guilty of enslaving its own people. But in course of his journey, it is not the slavery but the deplorable condition of public health that turns out to be real problem plaguing the country.

The beginning of Greene's journey is marked by the typical imperial fear of tropical diseases. He refers to what he read in the British Government's Blue Book and it describes Liberia to be a disease-hub –

> The absence of any attempt by the Government, not only to take effective steps to control yellow fever or plague, but even to arrange for the notification of yellow fever, as well as the complete lack of medical supervision of ships touching the Liberian coast...
>
> The great majority of the mosquito caught in Monrovia are of a species known to carry yellow fever...
>
> As far as is known, the principal diseases in the interior include elephantiasis, leprosy, yaws, malaria, hookworm, schistosomiasis, dysentery, smallpox and nutritional conditions. In the whole country there are only: two doctors in Monrovia, both foreign and both engaged in private practice, a medical officer on the Firestone Plantations, and three or four missionary doctors working in the interior...
>
> In Monrovia itself malaria is practically universal...
>
> (Greene 1980, 17-18)

In the second chapter (The Cargo Ship) this fear becomes more obvious when Greene introduces us with the fellow travellers–

> My cousin and I had five fellow passengers in the cargo ship: two shipping agents, a traveller for an engineering firm, a doctor on his way to the Coast with anti-yellow-fever serum, and a woman joining her husband at Bathurst. All except the woman and the traveller knew the Coast; they knew the same people; they had a common technique of living enforced by common conditions. The daily dose of quinine, mosquito-netting over all the pot-holes: these to them were as natural as the table-cloth at meals. (Greene1980, 23)

Greene's ironic observation, "One could begin a conversation with religion, politics, books; it always ended with malaria, plague, yellow fever" (Greene 1980, 24), sums up well the reality of diseases of the place towards which he is heading. These anticipations are to be evolved into lived experiences as he advances into the interiors of the country where disease becomes the panorama of intensified human suffering.

Cedric Watts in his book, *A Preface to Greene* emphasises Greene's medical humanistic zeal in *Journey without Maps*—

> Its best feature is probably the intense and discriminating interest that Greene took in the diversity of Africans whom he encountered, particularly in his considerate treatment of the various carriers and his compassionate concern for the suffering he observed. (Watts 1997, 35)

Actually in the interiors Greene comes closer to the ground reality of tropical diseases and people's utter helplessness in the absence of proper medication.

In many small towns and villages in the interior Greene came across a civilization where flies, mosquitoes and rats dominate and people live dangerously on the edge of their existence. In the night Greene mostly remained sleepless due to the extreme heat and free and uninhibited movements of mosquitoes, rats and flies around his bed. In Duogobmai, a town of the Buzie community, Greene is stupified by the immensity of the diseases and dirt. He says-

> The thought of disease began to weigh on my mind; I seemed to swallow it in the dust which soon inflamed my throat; I couldn't forget where the dust had come from, from the dung and the bitches and the sores on the feet. (Greene 1980, 128-129)

Or,

> And lying awake and hearing the rats play among our boxes, couldn't help remembering, too, the list of diseases I had read in England: leprosy, yaws, smallpox... They were all, I felt certain, to be found in Duogobmai,

> and it was no comfort to know that leprosy was hardly at all contagious and that none of these diseases could be contagious and that none of these diseases could be transmitted by fleas in a rat's fur. One felt that even the dust in the cramped dirty town was poisonous, no less than fleas. (Greene 1980, 132)

Greene has time and again referred to the aura of exoticism around a white man in Liberia because by then many native Africans had no prior experience of seeing a man with white complexion. Again the suffering tribes often took the advent of a strange white man to their town to be good sign for much awaited healing and medication. The native carriers also looked up to Greene for help to get rid of their long hidden venereal diseases. Greene writes-

> It was assumed that I would always be glad to see them there, to attend to their wants even in the middle of a meal, giving them iodine or Epsom salts. At Zigita a leprous man from the town came, with the sellers, to be healed, standing dumbly, holding out his rotting hands. Passive misery had been stamped on his face for a long while, but he had seen the carriers take medicine from me and one could tell that behind the misery a spark of belief had been struck in miracles. It was no good destroying hope and admitting there was nothing I could do. I gave him a few tablets of boric acid to dissolve and bathe his hands with. (Greene 1980, 137)

At the same time, the cluelessness of people in front of diseases and lack of medicines brings Greene to the verge of that cardinal medical humanistic realization that finally helps him shirk off his inner imperial prejudices. It happens only when he himself falls ill with fever and can easily perceive the perspective of wretched death without proper medication. Greene writes-

> This, as I grew more tired and my health a little failed, seemed to be what I would chiefly remember as Africa: cockroaches eating our clothes, rats on the floor, dust in the throat, jiggers under the nails, ants fastening on the flesh. ... White or black, they were living here for a short while on

> the surface of the land, but Africa had the last say, and it said in the forms of rats and ants … (Greene 1980, 144)

This realization, so, leads Greene to treat the naive carriers with deep sores on their feet caused by long and incessant walk barefoot even when he is cardinally ill and immensely tired. With his little medical knowledge he tried drastically to integrate medical scientific spirit and medical humanistic spirit to cure them –

> The guinea-worm makes its way through any sore in the foot, going up as far as the knee. When the foot is afterwards put in water the worm spews its eggs into the water through the sore. The only way to deal with it in the absence of a doctor is to find its end like a thread of cotton and wind it out in a long unbroken length round a match-stick. If the worm breaks, the leg may fester. (Greene 1980, 157)

In *Journey without Maps,* Greene also has introduced some people who have responded to the humanistic spirit of medicines. Dr. Harley, "the Methodist medical missionary" (Greene 1980, 170) in Liberia has been serving the helpless patients there for ten years " cutting away pus from the huge swollen genitals, injecting for yaws, anointing for craw-craw, injecting two hundred natives a week for venereal disease" (Greene 1980, 170). But people like him are very rare in Liberia and the darkness of death and disease never fades away.

Greene also describes his own psychological changes after recovery. The depressed and suicidal writer of the initial days of the journey falls in love with life anew-

> I was discovering in myself a thing I thought I had never possessed: a love of life. (Greene 1980, 171)

Or,

> It was like a conversion, and I had never experienced a conversion before. ... I had been completely convinced of the beauty and desirability of the mere act of living. (Greene 1980, 213-214)

Although the scene changes to India of 1857, the utter helplessness of human beings in the face of disease and the need for an integration of medical scientific spirit and medical humanistic spirit are also the central concerns in J. G. Farrell's novel, *The Siege of Krishnapur* (1973). The novel, as I have already pointed out, dramatizes the siege of a remote North Indian British outpost during the Indian Mutiny. The novel shows and deciphers the British characters in India who are ostracized in the garrison trying to resist political challenge of the Sepoys and the physical challenge posed by the outbreak of cholera in the household. The novel is ostensibly a critique of British imperialism in India and shows the futility of the Victorian complacency about progress and advancement in India under colonial rule. The initial description of the British community in Krishnapur and in Calcutta leading a life of pantries, laundries, music rooms and ballrooms is meant to provide a glimpse of that upper-lipped complacency which succumbs to the fear of extinction in the hand of the Sepoys in no time. At the same time, all main characters come close to the cardinal truth that the exponents of the East India Company lived rather dangerously in India during the Indian Revolution of 1857. The Collector, an orthodox Victorian believer of progress, turns into a bitter man after the siege. The Magistrate has lost his vibrant and sentimental political ideas and Fleury transforms into a soldier from a youth of romantic and poet-like sensibilities. The horror of the four-month-long siege amidst constant threats of being sublimated either by bullets or by cholera, hapless deaths of fellow Britishers, starvation and aggravation represents the ground reality of the time in a lucid manner.

In *The Siege of Krishnapur* Farrell challenges the tendency of the colonial and medical narratives to portray the British presence in India to be immensely beneficial for overall progress and development, particularly in matters relating to medicine and health. The Indian Medical Service officers were especially baffled about cholera. Mark Harrison in his book, *Public Health in British India: Anglo-Indian Preventive Medicine 1859-1914 (1994)* writes—

> Before 1817, cholera had been confined to Lower Bengal, with sporadic outbreaks among the rural population, but not among European enclaves in towns, or in military stations. In the year, however, the disease spread outside its 'home' in Bengal to claim the lives of many thousands of Indians and Europeans in northern and eastern India, and, in the following years, in the presidencies of Bombay and Madras. ...the outbreak of what appeared to be a new disease -*epidemic* cholera - made a profound impression on Europeans, arousing more fear and interest than any other disease. In the wake of further outbreaks of the disease, debate raged over the causation of cholera and how best to prevent it.
>
> No disease was more important, and no disease so little understood, as the 'epidemic cholera'. Hindu literature referred only to cholera in its sporadic, endemic form, while European practitioners conjectured variously that the disease was caused by the electrical state of the atmosphere; by the operation of climate on the soil, providing the right conditions for the germination of the cholera 'seed'; by contagion; or by transmission of the cholera germ in water (Snow's theory). Such questions acquired a fresh relevance after the mutiny, during which British troops had been seriously depleted by the disease. (Harrison 1994, 99)

This debate related to miasma and waterborne transmission of cholera between two doctors, Dr. Dunstaple and Dr. McNab questions the authoritative Victorian attitude of the colonial rulers who cannot avert diseases with all their so-called progress in medicines. Again continuous references to phrenology in the novel cast a cynical look upon that authority. Actually, before writing this novel Farrell had gone for an extensive research on the late 19th century medical history of colonial India. Here from the vantage point of the 1970s he looks back to the colonial past of his country. Malcolm Dean says that he found 19th century copies of the *British Medical Journal* among Farrell's papers which indicate the hard work he put to portray the medical condition in colonial India in a period-specific way.

Among the natural examples of scurvy, malnutrition, amputation and nervous breakdown that plague the British enclave in Krishnapur, the two main subjects that largely feature in Farrell's medical discourse are that of cholera and phrenology. The inclusion of infectious disease and pseudoscience is closely related to his concerns with medical humanism to a great extent. When cholera befalls the garrison, the first reaction to it was that of a confused fear because the old doctor, Dr. Dunstaple, who believes in the miasma theory relies mainly upon the Indian pseudoscience for the treatment of it. When one of the first cases of cholera is reported, Dunstaple is all ready to establish the authenticity of his theory by belittling Dr. McNab who is young and believes in the waterborne theory of cholera treating the patients with medicines and injection of saline water to avert dehydration. When the Collector himself becomes ill, Dunstaple becomes so enraged over McNab's methods that—

> Suddenly, he seized the Collector's wrist and dragged him across the ward to a mattress on which, pale as milk beneath a cloud of flies, a gaunt man lay shivering, stark naked.
>
> 'He's now in the consecutive fever... How d'you think I cured this man? How d'you think I saved his life?'
>
> The Collector offered no suggestion so the Doctor explained that he had used the best treatment known to medical science, the way he had been taught as a student, the treatment of which, for want of a specific, every physician worthy of the name accorded his cholera patients... calomel, opium and poultices, together with brandy as a stimulant. Every half hour he gave pills of calomel (half a grain), opium and capsicum (of each one-eighth of a grain). Calomel, the Collector probably didn't know, was an admirable aperient for cleansing the upper intestinal canal of morbid cholera poison. At the same time, to relieve the cramps he had applied flannels wrung out of hot water and sprinkled with chloroform or turpentine to the feet, legs, stomach and chest, and even to hands and arms. Then he had replaced them with flannels spread with mustard as his dispensers were now doing... At this point the Doctor tried to pull the Collector to yet another bed, where a Eurasian orderly was spreading

> mustard thickly with a knife on the chest and stomach of yet another tossing, groaning figure. But the Collector could stand no more and, shaking himself free, made for the door with the Doctor in pursuit. (Farrell 1993, 165-166)

What Dunstaple was doing is nothing more than mere quackery and making full use of his revered position among the people of Krishnapur he repeatedly calls McNab to prove his point that cholera is waterborne. But Dunstaple himself falls a prey to cholera when he allegedly swallowed a bottle of rice-water discharge gathered from a cholera patient in a bid to disprove McNab once and for all. Dunstaple sticks to his belief in the treatment of cholera and "...he had protested again and again, 'On no account let that charlatan near me'" (Farrell 1993, 270). His condition deteriorates and finally improves when McNab comes and injects him with Saline water. But he angrily refuses to undergo his treatment and soon dies. His death proves the emptiness of Victorian complacency about the advancement of medical science.

By the end of the novel, Farrell has presented a terrifying picture of the British community at Krishnapur who are reduced to eating dogs, horses and even beetles with their scurvy-loosened teeth as cholera, starvation and the sepoys have killed off most of the inmates. The utter helplessness of human beings in the face of physical destitution has been brilliantly depicted by Farrell here.

Again, another medical thread runs alongside the mounting tension over the treatment of cholera in the novel and that particular thread is phrenology. Mr. Willoughby, the Magistrate is the greatest proponent of phrenology in the novel. It is another European import to India and had been used as a classificatory discourse to catalogue "criminal tribes" (James 2007, 202). The Magistrate's intention of knowing the real characters of his fellow British people and the Indians alike by the patterns of their skulls has been wittily described by Farrell. Especially the episode where the Magistrate inspects the body of Miss Lucy Hughes, the so called fallen woman of the cantonment, is both funny and satirical. These pseudo-scientific practices, in the words of Sam Goodman, "like cholera, becomes a similarly vital means by which Farrell is able to illustrate the manner in which outdated medical ideas were able to retain a degree of professional cachet in the colonial setting long after their abandonment in European medical discourses" (Goodman 2015, 156).

Therefore, like Greene, Farrell is also concerned with the suffering that diseases engender and refers to the medical humanistic need to provide psychological support to the patient. Farrell himself died at the age of 44 and was partially disabled as a lasting effect of polio. In the words of John McLeod "illness and consequences are prevailing issues" (McLeod 2007, 5) in his novels. *The Siege of Krishnapur* shows that "British experience of India was intensely physical" (Collingham 2001, 1).

REFERENCES

Collingham, E. M. 2001. *Imperial Bodies.* Cambridge: Polity Press.

Farrell, J.G. (First Pub. 1973) 1993. *The Siege of Krishnapur.* London: Phoenix.

Gong, Fuquing, Yunpeng Diao, Taowen Pan, Min Liu, Hongliang Sun. 2015. "Evolution of Human Medical Model and Development Course of Medical Humanistic Spirit."*Biomedical Research* 26. No. 3. 407-414.

Goodman, Sam. 2015. "'A Great Beneficial Disease': Colonial Medicine and Imperial Authority in J. G. Farrell's *The Siege of Krishnapur.*" *The Journal of Medical Humanities* 36, No. 2: 141-156.

Greene, Graham. (First Pub. 1936) 1980. *Journey without Maps.* London: Penguin Books.

Harrison, Mark. 1994. *Public health in British India: Anglo-Indian preventive medicine 1859-1914.* Cambridge: Cambridge University Press.

James, Lawrence. 2007. *Raj: The Making and Unmasking of British India.* London: Abacus.

McLeod, J. 2007. *J. G. Farrell.* Hornden: Northcote House Publishers.

Watts, Cedric. 1997. *A Preface to Greene.* New Delhi: Pearson Education.

PART 3.
HISTORICAL CASE-STUDIES

In: Imperial Maladies
Editors: D. Bandyopadhyay et al.
ISBN: 978-1-53611-863-6

Chapter 8

The Curious Discourse of Mesmerism in Colonial Bengal - James Esdaile: A Case-Study

Shreya Chakravorty*
Department of English, Budge Budge College, Kolkata,
West Bengal, India

Introduction

Colonial history of medicine is a complex site of various conflicting and complementary modes of knowledge. Colonial Bengal, especially in the later half of the nineteenth century, is indeed a rich topos to study the dynamics between Western modes of scientific and often pseudo-scientific cures and their local counterparts - modes of healing that had existed as indigenous practices since time immemorial. James Esdaile (1808-1859), the first official practitioner of mesmerism as an anaesthetic agent during

* Corresponding author's address: Budge Budge College, 7 Deshabandhu Chittaranjan Rd., Budge Budge, South 24 Parganas, West Bengal, India. PIN: Kolkata-700137. Email: thisisonni@ gmail.com.

surgeries in Colonial Bengal is an interesting case-study in showing the complex correlation between Western and indigenous modes of healing.

After being appointed to India as an Assistant Surgeon to the East India Company in 1830, it took Esdaile fifteen years to perform his first mesmeric procedure. This gap was mainly owing to his sickness which saw him go back to England on an extended furlough. Ironically enough, the same time-period must have proved life-changing for Esdaile. It was during this period that John Elliotson, the celebrated British physician was incorporating a substantial section on Mesmerism in the fifth edition of his book *Human Physiology* (to be published in 1840). Mesmerism was showing promises of gaining ratification and sanction from the medical hierarchy for being advocated and championed by one of the pioneers of British medical science. No wonder then, that James Esdaile who came back to India was extremely hopeful and willing to incorporate mesmerism as a mode of treatment in the Indian colony where accountability for testing a new mode of treatment on a feeble and ill-nourished race would be much less compared to England. The constraints under which Elliotson had to work in England were almost non-existent for Esdaile in the Indian colony. That is the reason behind his direct incorporation of mesmerism as a surgical tool in Hooghly Imambara and Jail hospitals.

Throughout his career in India, Esdaile had performed numerous surgeries with the help of Mesmserism and had even attempted to alleviate mental disorders with the help of mesmeric trance. In fact, in a bid to gain recognition for mesmerism, he had written two books on the subject; namely, *Mesmerism in India and its Practical Application in Surgery and Medicine* (1847) and *Natural and Mesmeric Clairvoyance with the Practical Application of Mesmerism in Surgery and Medicine* (1852). This paper attempts to deal with Esdaile's complicated stance towards mesmerism in the first book entitled *Mesmerism in India and its Practical Application in Surgery and Medicine* (1847).

In *Mesmerism in India and its Practical Application in Surgery and Medicine*, in the very dedicatory epistle addressed to his father Rev. James Esdaile dated 1st February 1846, Dr. James Esdaile states, "However new and strange the subject of this work may be to you, I am sure that it will afford you pleasure to know that I have introduced, and… I may say established, a new and powerful means of alleviating human suffering among the natives of Bengal" (No page number given). Esdaile is rather adopting a messiah-like benevolent tone here which goes a long way in betraying his colonising urge. At this point he is perhaps hopeful about the status of mesmerism. He seems to be expecting that mesmerism will be included within the folds of institutional medicine in India because of his practical demonstration of its efficacy. Esdaile is in fact expecting the inclusion of mesmerism in the infinitely better western/colonial curative machinery in the long run.

In the 'Preface' dated the same as the dedicatory letter, Esdaile continues to speak in a similarly generous tone and begs to be allowed to demonstrate "the singular and most beneficial influence that mesmerism exerts over the constitution of the people of Bengal" (No page number given). He declares his profound belief in the fact that "painless surgical operations, and other medical advantages, are their natural birthright… of which" he hopes "they will be no longer deprived." When, on the one hand, mesmerism is being almost decidedly banned entrance into proper institutional medicine in England post 1838, Esdaile is seeking affirmation for the same practice in India by validating his research on the cumulative reports of its success on a considerable sample size of the native population. Perhaps he hoped to ascribe to mesmerism the honor of being called a properly scientific discipline by validating it first in the colonial laboratory.

The 'Preface' ends with the declaration of his forthcoming journey to join the army of the Sutlej in the capacity of a civil surgeon. He emphatically states that he hopes "to work out this curious subject in all its practical bearings, and to live to communicate" his experience to the public from there. But we never come across any such account. Whether he wrote anything substantial at all during his tenure at the Sutlej is not known. But, the conviction of Esdaile's declaration is incongruous with the absolute lack of output. As such, any attempt at a deliberate erasure of a medical treatise written by him based on his Sutlej experience cannot be completely ruled out either.

This prefatory letter is directly followed by a ceremonious introduction by James Esdaile's brother, Reverend David Esdaile. At the very outset of this section, David states that his brother had announced about his discovery of "something to dispel the *ennui* of Indian life, and that his mission was to become 'the Apostle of Mesmerism in India.' He confessed that his attention was grabbed by the manifestations of this incomprehensible power more than twelve years ago while reading an account given by M. Cloquet about removal of a cancerous breast under the influence of mesmeric trance. From that hour, he started believing that "many things, scouted by most people as frauds or delusions, were merely new manifestations of this incomprehensible power." Incredulity seemed irrational in the face of a plethora of evidence.

David further stated that the book written by his brother upon an imperfectly understood branch of science can be either categorised as a "literary performance" or a "philosophical treatise." It is extremely intriguing to see a book chiefly based on the medical account of various surgeries performed under mesmeric influence seeking justification as a "literary performance." This probably hints at the fluid nature of disciplines in the Colonial/Victorian academic hierarchy. It may further hint at the wobbling nature of identity of a nascent curative mechanism which wanted to gain admission into the sphere of institutional medicine through the buffer of literature.

David hoped that this book would help the British public in procuring information and perhaps restore their lost faith in the so-called "derided science" of mesmerism. After this, he presents the prospective reading public with an unusual justification for exploring the mesmeric practice. He argues, fallen in wrong hands, mesmerism can wield a tremendously nefarious influence, especially in a country like India where detestable crimes are rampant. Therefore, in order to prevent crimes with the help of the mesmeric tool, legislators must declare its practice penal except by regularly educated medical men. In this section of the Preface, the predominant tone of the author is premonitory and full of caution. David believes "it (mesmerism) is a most formidable source of mischief in the hands of the ignorant and the unprincipled." It is, as if, he seeks defense for his brother's work on the ethical ground of saving the gullible, almost illiterate colonised from these distorted practitioners of the mesmeric art.

However, his brother Dr. Esdaile makes way for a rather rational opening fit for a medical practitioner. In the very opening of his book, he exhorts his readership to effect a paradigmatic shift in their mode of thinking by rejecting the "respectable" old notion that "the vital powers of our bodies are confined within their own limits, and cannot be transferred to and act upon others." On the contrary, there is sufficient ground to suppose that "the vital fluid of one person can be poured into the system of another." Man is not confined within the pent-house of his body. "A merciful God has ingrafted a communicable, life-giving curative power in the human body, in order that when two individuals are found together, deprived of the aids of art, the one in health may often be able to soothe and relieve his sick companion, by imparting to him a portion of his vitality" (Esdaile 1847, 28). In a typical medical treatise, Esdaile uses God as an alibi to account for man's innate, inexplicable spiritual power enriched with healing properties.

Esdaile urges common readership, not the medical fraternity, to develop a mentality of rational acceptance of apparently inexplicable phenomenon, if and only if supported by evidence. He takes the reverse route; that is, he wants sanctification of the mesmeric practice and its admission into the Pharmacopoeia as the culmination of the large-scale support by ordinary colonial Indians. He rather cautions that if general public depends on doctors to ratify this curative practice for them, "… not many of this generation will live to benefit by Mesmerism" (Esdaile 1847, 32).

He thereby categorically recommends the public to exercise their common sense and sober judgment in determining for the doctors that Mesmerism is a remedial method of great efficacy; that lack of knowledge about this nascent method is a matter of discredit for medical men. Common men will coax the medical fraternity into acceptance of Mesmerism as a remedial agent. But only after the practitioners of institutional medicine ratify Mesmerism as a valid curative method, "will it (Mesmerism) assume its proper rank."… "and be lodged in the hands of those who should alone practice it…" (Esdaile 1847, 33). Mesmerism is a tremendously powerful method of exerting influence over others which can wield devastatingly negative impact on vulnerable targets, if abused. If it gets institutional sanction, punishment for offenders will also be formulated with equal strictness. This will result in lowering the level of abuse of Mesmerism by people with wicked intentions.

It is by medical men of India that, Esdaile believes, the truth or falsehood of Mesmerism be speedily decided since they are the means of putting in motion a law of nature whose springs are hidden from common people but whose effects are most wonderful and beneficial to humanity when properly channelised. He continues stating how tedious and laborious it is to induce in people a trance approximating a comatose state of complete insensibility. But the mesmeriser must strive to achieve it. Once he decodes the secret behind induction of successful mesmeric trance, "all is easy, for any number of proper assistants may be taught to act under our superintendence" (Esdaile 1847, 35). It is rather interesting to find out that Esdaile practiced exactly what he preached. After a very brief, initial stint of inducing mesmeric trance in patients himself, he vested this responsibility upon his assistants. He only took care of the surgical section of the entire procedure.

Esdaile then tries to draw the portrait of an ideal mesmeriser. He believes that mesmerisers cannot be convinced into becoming one, rather they should follow the example of successful predecessors and take up the art willingly. Esdaile says that it is unfair to enumerate the physical and moral qualities of a mesmeriser and one must be deterred from the attempt to paint the picture of a 'perfect monster' in his name. The ideal mesmeriser, however, should be endowed with certain physical traits. He should have strong and equally agile nervous and circulating systems. He must also possess a determined will and "a resolution to do the thing if possible." His love for truth and humanity would induce him to "do for love what gold could never buy" (Esdaile 1847, 35). We cannot but continue to observe the tone of benevolence permeating the trope of 'coloniser-mesmeriser.' A threat lingers in the wings, the uncanny potential of 'mock-magnanimity' informing the entire scope or connotation of the term 'mesmeriser.'

A little down the line, Esdaile starts recapitulating his experience as a mesmerizer. He confesses that he found the act of inducing mesmeric trance in his patients extremely hectic and exhausting. Consequently, he started initiating his assistants into the art of mesmerism, he justifies. These "young Hindoos and Mahomedans" became skilful mesmerisers in almost no time. Such was the success of Esdaile - the teacher of the art of mesmerism, that a dozen assistants became ready to execute his wishes, "whether it be in the mesmeric treatment of medical cases, or for procuring coma in surgical operations" (Esdaile 1847, 36).

For those who want to venture into the territory of mesmerism through self-learning be better guided by an earnest desire to know the truth, a fixed attention and a resolution to overcome difficulties, warns Esdaile. First, experiments should be conducted on the sick in the hope of genuinely benefitting them. He further cautions his readers or aspiring mesmeris ers that they must not experiment on healthy subjects who are very difficult as mesmerisees. He argues "The whole need not a physician, but they that are sick" (Esdaile 1847, 36). Bountiful nature never wastes her resources unnecessarily.

If the medicine of nature or mesmerism is forcefully applied upon healthy individuals, it is very likely to do mischief. Any attempt to stay better than well will surely make one sick, according to Esdaile. But even such a confident exponent of the mesmeric art seems to be unsure on a vital issue. He cannot pronounce which person can, most definitely, be brought under mesmeric influence. He has to try his hand at him or her before realising his client's capacity to be mesmerised. Yet, he states resolutely that most of the patients that he and his assistants have handled in the mesmeric hospital have been successfully mesmerised; few cases where mesmeric trance could not be induced could also have become successful, if only handled with a little more perseverance.

It is just at the beginning of the first chapter of his lengthy treatise on the efficacy of mesmerism that Esdaile has already expounded his stance. He has projected himself as a serious dabbler in this art. He has already stated in unequivocal terms that he wants to expound the prospects and consequences of practising this art in the largest British colony called India.

But his benevolent tone betrays an element of condescension which will become clear in course of the same chapter. In course of expounding the benefits of mesmerism, Esdaile further states that in contrast to the Europeans, the Indian race has a natural proclivity towards surrendering to mesmeric manipulations since "a depressed state of the nervous system favours its reception." His opinion on the population of Bengal, even if pitted in the 1840s, shows nothing more than the retrogressive and explicit racism of a European medical practitioner. According to him, the Bengal population is "a feeble, ill-nourished race, remarkably deficient in nervous energy" (Esdaile 1847, 37), whose natural debility of constitution is lowered still by disease. Yet, these constitutional drawbacks are congenial to the induction of mesmeric trance, a higher susceptibility quotient increasing the possibility of being successfully cured; especially if an equally susceptible mental constitution complements this physical feebleness. Unlike Europeans, Indians do not exhibit a "morbid irritability of nerves, and the mental impatience of the civilized man." At and from this point, Esdaile suddenly changes his tone. He adopts a typical Rousseauvian stance and compares the native with a "noble savage" unadulterated by the machinations of civilisation. He changes quarters and lauds Indians for the very same qualities that he found derogatory a few lines back. He expresses relief in not having to "contend against" the civilised man and his baggage of knowledge before making the naïve native surrender to the will of nature that prevails through mesmerism. His success, he believes, is mainly owing to his patients, the "simple unsophisticated children of nature" who do not think, question or remonstrate. Here is an interesting divide within the humanistic and enlightened European mode of consciousness. An educated section of the custodians of rationality think that it is easier to impose experimental modes of medicinal cure upon an unassuming native population to whom they are no less than demi-gods. But, it is rather difficult to prove the authenticity of their analgesic technique to their co-brethren steeped and bathed in the lore of rationality. Nature has rejected the artificial orientation of the European constitution and left her European children to their "hallowed" self-sufficiency. But their make-shifts and palliatives are nothing in comparison with the steady and curative powers of enduring nature. The true physician tries to induce the flow of energy from nature to the diseased agent ultimately aiming at removing any impediments in the way of establishing such a rapport. But the average artificial practitioner of medical science would "rarely condescend to divide with nature the merit of the cure" (Esdaile 1847, 39). He would attribute his success to himself first and then to his pills and powders. Anyone who affects cure by hailing the unassisted powers of nature would be instantly dubbed by him as a "quack, imposter, or fool, and hunted down as a *fera naturae*" (Esdaile 1847, 39).

The implication of this last legal term is far-reaching and loaded with resonances in the context of colonial domination. The 'fera/ferae naturae' is a wild soul with the vulnerability of being trapped, tortured and dominated by another; it merely replicates the subaltern position of the native colonised whereby the idiom of domination becomes equivalent to the legal right of the white, superior coloniser. Esdaile ends up suggesting that even the hardly socially amenable colonised have the proclivity of being legally dominated to the point of being exploited by the coloniser. Any amount of native inclination towards establishing a liaison with nature in a bid to heal is treated as nothing less than "ec-centricity." This section betrays a subtle hint that the coloniser has the right to declare an ingeniously armed mesmerist as "wild" in the sense of being an "outcast" even while retaining the power to judge or exploit his art of healing. In any case, Esdaile is strictly against such an exclusionist attitude of the western medical fraternity. He even quotes Hippocrates to justify his advocacy of mesmeric treatment thus: "Nothing should be omitted in an art which interests the whole world, which may be beneficial to suffering humanity, and which does not risk human life and comfort" (Esdaile 1847, 39). Esdaile in fact challenges institutionalised medicinal practice by indicating the possibility of an alternative method of natural therapy whereby men must study the sources of natural remedy – resources which sustained humanity much before the discovery of pills and potions.

In the next section, Esdaile attempts to prove that mesmerism is the oldest and most natural mode of curing many of the severe, "uncomplicated" diseases of the human race. The curative power of this method was known to "savages" before the advent of sobering civilisation. Among the savage races, conjurers practiced this art by skillfully concealing the secret of their power by incantations or mummery. Interestingly enough, Esdaile suspects that in most cases, the so-called quacks affected miraculous acts of healing without even knowing animal magnetism to be the reason behind this cure. He reinstates his belief in the presence of this practice in India since time immemorial "like every other custom in this immutable society" (Esdaile 1847, 43). In fact, he quotes at length from his own "Mesmeric Journal" to prove his point even further. In his journal entry dated 9th June, 1845, he states having had the good fortune of being introduced to one of the most famous magicians of Bengal. The native magician was appointed for treating a patient of hysteria but Esdaile had done his wonders on her till the Indian magician arrived. However, Esdaile got introduced to this magician as a "brother magician who had studied the art of magic in different parts of the world, but particularly in Egypt, where I had learnt the secrets of the great Sooleyman from the moollahs and fuqueers" (Esdaile 1847, 43). Such an intimidating and forced introduction would have created a recoiling effect. No wonder, when Esdaile asserted his desire to ascertain whether their charms were the same, the native magician was difficult to be persuaded. He probably agreed to show Esdaile his process for assuaging pain only after Esdaile asserted how "the hakeems of Europe held the wise men of the east in high estimation, knowing that all knowledge had come from that quarter" (Esdaile 1847, 43). Esdaile is asserting his supremacy as a magician by showing off his hold over oriental knowledge and trying to coax the native magician into action by glibly praising oriental wisdom as the most authentic and original source of knowledge. But very soon, in course of the same section of the book we find that all this praise is a prologue to establishing his own supremacy as a far better, knowledgeable and trained mesmeriser in comparison with his ignorant "brother magician" (Esdaile 1847, 43). The native mesmeriser's administration of mesmerised water with a twig over the paining body of the patient is at best an ill-informed endeavor at affecting analgesic cure. The exerciser of this move is hardly aware of the force operating behind this apparently inexplicable and magical cure.

However, Esdaile pretends to be convinced by the efficacy of the native mesmeriser's charms in alleviating pain just to show the greater effectiveness of his own scientific moves in due course. He even gains the confidence of this naïve native by ceremoniously chanting the chorus of "King of the Cannibal Islands" before sending him into a mesmeric trance. The reiteration of the trope of Africa as the seat of magic and miracle, first with the assertion of the source of his magical knowledge to be ancient Egypt and then by chanting this song shows two aspects. Firstly, Esdaile is taking advantage of his position as a coloniser with exposure to institutional medicinal knowledge. He is doing it without showing the least amount of respect towards this native magician whom he infantilises and demeans at his own will. Secondly, ironically enough, he is trying to gain the confidence of this native practitioner of mesmeric art not by resorting to his superior repertoire of knowledge but by a mocking reference to a much revered ancient tradition of miraculous healing located outside continental Europe. Esdaile proceeds further to describe his casting of a mesmeric spell upon this magician in spite of the latter's utmost defensive efforts to ward off the same. Esdaile continues to describe his successful casting of the spell, "I was sure that I had caught my brother magician napping, but, in a few minutes, he bolted up suddenly, clapped his hands to his head, cried he felt drunk, and nothing could induce him to lie down again; *abiit, excessit, evasit, erupit*" (Esdaile 1847, 44). But very soon Esdaile realises that the native magician had fled in the fear of being completely mesmerised by him. On the occasion of their next meeting when Esdaile tries to concede his own defeat by saying "Well, you were too strong for my charm last night, I could not put you to sleep," the magician says "Oh! Yes, Sahib," "you did; I allow it; it is allowed that you put me to sleep" (Esdaile 1847, 44). This last statement by the native magician is loaded with implications that any postcolonial critique would try to dissect and analyse. The magician is either referring to the technical term of "allowing" the mesmeriser to cast spell over his mesmerisee – that moment of achieving a mindset of complete vulnerability in front of the mesmeriser by the would-be mesmerised. It is a difficult psycho-somatic state for a man with strong nerves to achieve, especially for someone who is an adept in casting spells over others and holds a subjective status (in being independent, not in the sense of being the subject). Or, the native magician is referring to the classic colonial binary of exploitation and justification of such manipulation by resorting to the quasi-divine authority of the coloniser which grants him universal allowance within the colonised space.

His position as a coloniser becomes prominent when he betrays an enlightened self-interest in seeking to defend the native origin of mesmeric art. It is proved beyond any doubt to Esdaile that the practice of mesmerism had been known to the countrymen since ages. In a few cases, while administering mesmeric passes, his patients confessed having met similar modes of treatment in the past from Indian hakims, only that the process had some other name. Esdaile writes, "It thus appears that the beneficial effects of the mesmeric processes are known in this country, and the secret has probably descended from remote antiquity, in certain families or castes" (Esdaile 1847, 45). Esdaile further shows his growing concern on discovering the nefarious ends to which the art of somnambulism has been used in India. The fact that somnambulism has been used "for the most villainous purposes" is enough to prove that Indians apply mesmerism for achieving positive as well as negative ends. This evil propensity of mesmerism has been one of the most favorite objections raised against its formal introduction as a method of medicinal cure. Yet, at that point, the evidence of its existence and power could no longer be resisted according to Esdaile.

The tendency of all power depends upon the direction to which it is used, that is, the nature of power is determined by the end to which it is either wielded or judiciously administered. Just as opium, mercury or prussic acid can be used for negative purposes without the risk of being excluded from the pharmacopoeia, mesmerism should be given a fair chance in spite of its known propensity for being used to achieve hideous ends.

In fact, publicity is the biggest security against the manipulation of mesmeric powers for achieving nefarious ends. Esdaile states, "That this agent may, and will, be turned to the most diabolical purposes, is most certain, if the public will not be at the trouble to think upon the subject, and defend itself by common sense precautions" (Esdaile 1847, 46). Common people should know how to separate the grain from the chaff. They must realise that "the abuse, and not the use of any great power, is to be dreaded and guarded against" (Esdaile 1847, 46).

At this point, Esdaile makes a very vital, if not the most important statement of his thesis. He proposes to treat mesmerism, not as a psycho-somatic, but as a purely physical mode of healing. He hopes to prove through his experiments that the separate regions of the mind and body have been unnecessarily and perplexingly intermingled by former mesmeric observers; that they can be treated separately while administering mesmeric cure. This will not only simplify the mesmeric treatment of the disease, but remove the principal objection against it; namely – the necessity of often acting injuriously upon the mind while attempting to cure a physical ailment. He assures his readers that he has never attempted to influence the mind through his practice of mesmerism. Never, even for once, has he established mental "rapport" with his patients while administering mesmeric passes. Administering mesmerism for the purpose of affecting mental cure is just an additional advantage that this method can offer, an "extension of blessing" as Esdaile calls it, and should be exercised with tremendous caution. He asserts confidently, "I am convinced that in the majority of bodily evils removable by this means, there will be no need to interfere with the mind at all" (Esdaile 1847, 47). Why should one travel out of record? In case a mesmeric treatment combining physical and mental is required, it can be safely adopted by asking an honest man with the necessary knowledge. "Many will be disappointed that I have no mental wonders to relate" he continues, "My researches have been purely physical, and preclude me from getting at the mind at all, for all activity of the mind is the natural enemy of the purely physical impressions made upon the system" (Esdaile 1847, 47). He uses this method only for treating acute diseases and for inducing insensibility to pain. He could also have deployed it as a mental phenomenon in case so required. But his principal object being alleviation of physical suffering, he has deliberately withheld venturing into the troubled sea of metaphysics. All his efforts have been concentrated upon solving the more pressing bodily problems till a "terra firma" of indisputable facts is created from where the higher mysterious regions of the mind can be safely ventured into when and if required.

Hereafter, Esdaile puts foreword another argument against venturing into the "metaphysical" aspect of mesmerism. Administering mesmeric passes for alleviating physical pain is easier on his patients who belong to the poorest and most ignorant set of people on earth, Physique wise, men are similar world over: "a universal vital law reduces all to the same level of animal" (Esdaile 1847, 48). Even a coolie can mesmerise a philosopher for reducing his physical pain. But in order to affect someone at the level of mind through mesmerism, there needs to exist a kind of empathy which is impossible to achieve by the Western educated man in case of his native patients. The difference of morale between the European man and his native subjects is so great that it amounts to "actual antipathy and mutual repulsion" (Esdaile 1847, 48). Fine mental sympathy or rapport can be elicited in higher mental phenomenon; it might even be necessary. But Esdaile confesses, "my patients and I have probably too little in common to admit of mental sympathy between us" (Esdaile 1847, 49). Yet, he claims to have created a "singular bouleversement" in the minds of coolies and pariahs or outcastes when under the mesmeric influence. "Bouleversement" means "a reversal" or "violent disturbance" or "disorder."

Two aspects deserve special attention here: Firstly, Esdaile claims to have avoided building up mental rapport with his patients since the huge difference of morale between the Western man and the native can hardly be bridged, if at all. Then, why did he shy away from mesmerising his native patients even when trying to anaesthetise them before surgery? A surgery is supposed to begin and end with the body without any intervention into the mental realm. But he did not mesmerise his patients on his own. He always deployed native mesmerisers – young Hindus and Muslims for the purpose of inducing trance among his native and not-so-illustrious patients. Does that not indicate a presupposition on Esdaile's part of the inevitibility of establishing a mental rapport with his patients even while mesmerising them prior to a surgery (and not for curing any mental disease like hysteria or epilepsy)? A mental rapport would always be built up, one mind had to take reins over another mind - whether the patient needed to be mesmerised for analgesic purposes or to be rescued from a certain mental instability. In spite of his professions to the contrary, Esdaile could never disavow the inherently psychological nature of a mesmeric trance for whatever curative reasons it was used.

Secondly, though he reportedly refused to mesmerise because of the mental exhaustion induced by such a process, it does not require a drastic sweep of imagination to realise that the reason behind denial was more than skin-deep. He could probably not establish "rapport" with a much inferior native. Antipathy and repulsion would have been the two possible hindrances leading to failure in establishing a mesmeric bond. Possibility of failure must have intimidated Esdaile in attempting to build up a mental liaison with his native patients. No wonder, all he could build up in the name of a "rapport" with the natives was a "singular bouleversement (upheaval, not relief) in the minds of coolies and pariahs" (Esdaile 1847, 49), the best that a clash of two contrasting ideologies can gain if one attempts to supersede the other.

Before concluding these prefatory remarks he begs his reading audience, of which there is a substantial section of natives, not to commit the gross injustice of taking him for a mesmeric doctor, "for it would be as true to call me a rhubarb, jalap, or castor oil physician" (Esdaile 1847, 49). He claims to be deploying mesmerism as the last resort on patients on whom all other medicinal resources are exhausted and further begs his reading public to excuse any "unintentional mistakes" behind his assumptions. He venerates and debases at the same breath what he holds to be a revolutionary medical invention. He is hesitant about the reception of his thesis and is definitely trying to test the waters by adopting all suitable precautions.

Very soon, in the third chapter of this book, Esdaile attempts to seek validation for mesmerism yet again. But this time, he seeks validation by trying to find its roots in Europe. Esdaile begins this chapter by proclaiming emphatically that the effects produced by mesmerism were nearly as various as the different persons acted upon and "corresponded perfectly with the appearances observed in Europe…" (Esdaile 1847, 76). He rationalises further by saying that if the same effects follow the cause on the banks of the Thames, Seine, Rhine and Hooghly, it can be safely concluded that the same force is at work everywhere. He quotes Dupotet at length and refers to Deleuze's Practical Instructions to describe mesmeric sleep. He also makes passing references to Chenevix, Elliotson, Townshend and all other well-known mesmerists of the time to show that the conclusions he has reached about mesmeric sleep are exactly the same as these pioneers. He begs his readership "to compare my [his] account of Mesmerism in Bengal with this statement of its effects in Europe, and then say whether the identity of the thing in the east and west is not established:-" (Esdaile 1847, 77).

Through various case studies, Esdaile attempts to prove the universality of certain truths regarding mesmeric phenomena for advocating which a few honest and independent men have been laughed and scorned at from the end of eighteenth till the first half of the nineteenth century. Apart from the personal gratification acquired from finding entrance into nature's secret territory and finding the advantages of imitating her processes, Esdaile also believes it to be his noble responsibility to raise the "dishonoured dead" into public consideration and bestow respect due to them as benefactors of mankind. Esdaile expresses wonder at the relatively late realisation of England about the efficacy of mesmerism in comparison with its neighbour France. It is perhaps for the same reason that Esdaile wishes to base all his experiments in Calcutta and have Calcuttans, not Englishmen for his witnesses (not to forget the ancestry of this practice that he traces back to India).

Next, he uses the colonised space to defend himself against charges of possible fraudulence. He categorically states that it is morally impossible for him to influence his patients since he does not know any more about their symptoms than they do. He has gradually trained himself by observing each and every case, unique in its own right. Nature, not reason, has been his guide. He declares not to have read any book on mesmerism before treating his first patient. Adopting mesmeric means for inducing coma is also a circumstantial, not a premeditated decision and always adopted as a last resort. He emphasises upon the impossibility of his teaching the art of hiding pain to his patients. The horrific and unbearable pain of such surgical procedures can only be withstood through superhuman pain-containing power which is impossible for even persevering races as native Indians to perfect.

Esdaile is trying to base his case-studies on a purely colonial ground. He is more hopeful about the naïveté of native Indians, coolies and poor people of Calcutta, than the educated and skeptic population at home. He is trying to resuscitate a branch of so-called pseudo-scientific healing by taking recourse to its oriental bearings. Yet, he demeans the same population by showing their lack of awareness in practising this marvellous art of healing and benefitting by it, by showing how they brandish this natural art under the banner of mumbo-jumbo.

Further through this chapter, Esdaile repeatedly defends himself against accusations of imposture or faking of insensibility by his patients in the name of mesmeric trance. He presents many cases of severe surgical operations rendered possible only through introduction of mesmerism. In a bid to defend him to a desperate extent, Esdaile brings up two such surgical cases where even involuntary muscles like eye and thoracic muscles were rendered completely inactive because of induction of mesmeric trance.

On the whole, throughout this chapter, Esdaile is extremely eager to prove that mesmerism is not an act of imposture. It is extremely commendable on Esdaile's part to have tried to prove his point completely on the basis of observed facts in the presence of sceptical witnesses and not upon the slightest whiff of conjecture.

From the fourth chapter on, however, the absolutely verifiable and empirical nature of his observations veers slightly towards the subjective. In this chapter, Esdaile tries to investigate into the phenomenon of somnambulism and tries to make his patients attain this state of physically active trance through mesmerism. All of a sudden, Esdaile becomes witness to a case of alleged abduction of a ten to twelve year old boy by a barber. Esdaile recounts how he encountered a crowd of people in front of the "police office" while driving through Hooghly Bazaar. The boy was half dazed and sat on the lap of his rescuer with a swollen eye. The culprit was shown to Esdaile and in no time Esdaile investigated into the tools of this alleged barber and found his professional claim to be true. On recovering his senses, the boy narrated the tale of his abduction. He was sauntering in the field close to his home when this alleged abductor crossed the road, came up to him and started muttering charms. He took hold of the boy's hand and passed his hand across his eyes. The boy promptly lost his senses and followed the man, as if compelled by some invisible force. When he came to senses, he found himself outside the gates of Chandernagore, two miles away from his house. This little boy was not an imbecile and had never suffered from hysteric fits or sleep-walking problems. He had not eaten, drunk or smoked in the presence of this barber. Upon asking the barber, Esdaile got a completely different story where the barber himself pretended to be the rescuer. The two accounts given by two parties were completely dissimilar and if the boy's account was to be believed, Esdaile "could only see two roads out of the dilemma: it was either a case of natural or artificial somnambulism; and if the latter" he concluded "how could it be brought about unless by Mesmerism?" (Esdaile 1847, 99).

The trade of the alleged abductor roused suspicion in Esdaile and made him partial towards the boy's account. He claimed to have heard that barbers in India could put people to sleep while performing their tedious procedures. Also, there were various reports of people, all over India, who had been charmed out of their senses and obliged to follow their alleged charmers. Most importantly, in most of the cases, women were the victims of such somnambulistic trances. Till here, Esdaile seems to be giving an account of the predominance of somnambulism, possibly mesmeric, in the Indian sub-continent. But very soon, he goes on to generalise the mesmerising tendencies of the barbers world over, irrespective of their geographic location. He observes that all barbers are shrewd and observant. Their occupation brings them into close contact with those parts of the body which are easily susceptible to mesmeric influence. Therefore he concludes, "they are … very likely to have become possessed of the secret of Mesmerism at an early period, and perhaps it has descended to them as a mystery of their craft" (Esdaile 1847, 99). In case, he is called upon to bear witness, Esdaile wanted to make experiments to satisfy himself first. He thought if he had to assert that the evil barber has resorted to mesmerism to abduct the boy in the court of law, he should be able to produce somnambulistic trance through mesmeric experiments in his hospital in the first place. He was successful in producing somnambulistic trance from among his patients in the Jail hospital and put it up as the probable cause behind abduction. But Esdaile was asked to prove the veracity of his belief. "…the judge therefore asked me [him] if I [he] had any objection to show the Moulavies in court that it was possible for one person to make another follow him involuntarily…" (Esdaile 1847, 101). In two days' time, Esdaile was able to induce somnambulistic trance through mesmerism in two people, namely Nazir Mahomed and Sooroop Chand, in front of a court crowded with natives and Europeans. Esdaile was not as keen on trying to prove if the boy has been abducted mesmerically than he was eager to have an opportunity to publicly prove that somnambulistic trance can be induced through mesmerism.

From the moment Esdaile witnessed the extreme power of mesmerism, he became convinced of its power to do both good and evil. He harps on this point in his book to a considerable extent in the hope of rousing public awareness to a sense of the dangers as well as benefits that may be expected from mesmerism. He expresses his hope and trust that such an unbiased presentation of the plain and simple facts of mesmerism will help build up public opinion about it - whereby people will start strongly condemning those who practise this art for nefarious ends and applaud such efforts which tend to use mesmerism for philosophical and medical purposes. Finally, it was proved beyond any doubt that the barber was in illegal possession of the boy. He was even sentenced to nine years of rigorous imprisonment and labour in irons. This sentence was even confirmed by the superior court. But at this point, something unfortunate happens. Seeing that mesmeric experiments had made too deep an impression upon the court of law, government calls for the proceedings and surprisingly enough graciously pardons the barber. It is extremely surprising to see the sweep or universal hold of the British Government even over the judiciary which is supposed to be the highest authority for wielding justice. At this point, Esdaile sadly concludes upon the nature of human curiosity. He opines that instead of becoming "puzzled by the unexpected exhibition of new and wonderful bodily [sic] or mental phenomenon" (Esdaile 1847, 103) and denying or contemptuously dismissing them as the offspring of deception or delusion, man should try to come closer to truth by suspecting that they have overlooked some power of the human constitution. They should immediately take to the study of the nature of this new and apparently inexplicable reason rather than dismissing it summarily.

Up to this point, Esdaile's position is clear. He is trying to gain sanction for a relegated branch of healing by presenting numerous empirical instances and a few subjective, psychological proofs. But his argument takes a completely unpredictable turn in the last chapter. This chapter bears testimony to an unexpected, rather shocking change of position on behalf of the author. The same author who declares his resolution of keeping mind and body apart while conducting mesmeric treatment is finally and very unfortunately convinced into practising psychic feats through mesmerism. He opens the chapter with an elaborate justification that though his original intention was to confine himself strictly to an examination of the medical pretensions of mesmerism, he has been driven by the force of circumstances "out of the prudent mesmeric course" which he had decided to follow.

He claims that at the outset, his intention was to eschew all but the practical aspects of mesmerism in order to open the minds of men to receive new truths out of self-interest. But from this point he begins to change his position very cunningly. He says, "Not that I was, by any means, indifferent to the philosophie and extra-professional bearings of the subject…" (Esdaile 1847, 229). Let us be reminded that the same man had stated a few pages back in Chapter One of the same book that, "I am convinced that in the majority of bodily evils removable by this means, there will be no need to interfere with the mind at all" (Esdaile 1847, 47) and added that "Many will be disappointed that I have no mental wonders to relate" (Esdaile 1847, 47). Here he justifies his former stance by saying that he refrained from referring to the psychological impact of mesmerism in the first place because "the gross and palpable bodily phenomena, even, were more than the public stomach could bear" (Esdaile 1847, 229). He added that he did not serve up, on purpose, more than his reading public could digest at one go. This passage is that one stroke which instantly goes against the author and demolishes all that he had created so painstakingly and meticulously, in such detail, for so long. He confesses that his veering off course is accidental yet instrumental in determining his course of action which he had "resolved to follow (emphasis mine)" (Esdaile 1847, 229). At this point he even tries to hide behind the notions of Horatian "utile" and "dulce" by seeking prior justification for indulging in the latter (by dedicating a chapter to the "Curiosities of Mesmerism") since he has already dedicated a considerable part to the former.

In the next section, Esdaile asserts his aversion to public display of mesmeric skills. He is well aware, he claims, of the worthlessness of public exhibitions in convincing people towards the truth of mesmerism. He is "determined not to be made a showman of" (Esdaile 1847, 230). All performances of mesmeric skills are supposed to resort to artificial or fake means when nature does not cooperate at times. This unethical step is taken to procure success at the cost of truth. Moreover, the careful and intelligent observer does not have the necessary means of close inspection required to convince him. The entire act appears to be nothing more than "all humbug" (Esdaile 1847, 230) since it is beyond comprehension.

At this point in the book, Esdaile finally declares that it is absurd to set limits to any unexplored regions of nature. Esdaile claims to have acted with significant consistency in the preceding months in directing his "public" experiments towards purely professional subjects. But gradually, a general curiosity was excited in the public regarding this practice and he was at length requested from a high quarter to satisfy some of the inhabitants of Government-House with an especial mesmeric "Séance." Esdaile's opinion at this point is nothing short of being blasphemous to his entire lore of thought and experiments. He says, "This I could hardly have refused without appearing churlish" (Esdaile 1847, 230). A practising doctor employing mesmerism to alleviate pain of patients undergoing complicated surgeries now turns to mesmerism as a medium of communicating with the spirits of dead people. He consents to this request under another obligation. He is apprehensive of being accused of cowardice in case he does not consent to inspection during his own proceedings. He admits: "I therefore thought it best to submit to a necessary evil, and make the most of it, by converting an exclusive party into as general and promiscuous a meeting as possible" (Esdaile 1847, 230-31). It must be noted that the term "promiscuous" has not been used in its standard connotation of sexual profligacy but in the sense approximating 'individuals of different kinds brought together without order.' Esdaile aims at making this meeting a nodal point for various cross-sections of the society in order to convince as many people of the "magic" of mesmerism.

It is rather surprising to see that the same person who was visited by a medical committee in July 1846 in order to witness the efficacy of mesmerism as an analgesic in surgeries, is looking foreword to laymen's participation in mass-meetings to validate the super-sensory powers of mesmerism only a year back. Esdaile consents to exhibit the powers of mesmeric trance for non-professional purposes in 1845 in this meeting. But within a year's time, in July 1846, he seeks professional validation for the same practice by welcoming a medical committee to the Hooghly Imambara and Jail hospitals. It is highly intriguing that in this book that he publishes in 1847, he chooses to invert the chronological order of his experiences. He publishes his medical experiments with mesmerism before and goes ahead to depict the extra-sensory feats accomplished by mesmerism later. He offers the impossible to his audience only after preparing them through demonstrations of medical mesmerism over the past few months. But this time too Esdaile tries to seek validation for the wondrous workings of mesmerism by taking into confidence six medical men who belong to this huge crowd. Thereafter, Esdaile proceeds to quote at length from the newspaper to which one of the six members had testified regarding the veracity of the incidents reported. Under the title of "Public Display of Mesmerism at Hooghly" addressed "To the Editor of the *Englishman*," this man of science writes, "I esteem myself fortunate in having been present at an exhibition of powers of Mesmerism, given by Dr. Esdaile… to satisfy public curiosity, as it is the last opportunity of the kind likely to occur, Dr. E. having for this once only, consented to mesmerise for non-professional purposes" (Esdaile 1847, 231). In this meeting, Esdaile who proclaimed himself the prisoner of rationality had actually offered options to an eager audience whether they would prefer to see a woman made senseless by mesmerised water, or through the wall. The following section of this letter by the man of medicine almost reads like Dr. Elliotson's experiments on the O'Keys, though the nature of the latter experiments were bent more towards clairvoyance than somnambulism. According to the letter, on the same day, Esdaile conducts many other such experiments on prisoners to show the efficacy of mesmerism by inducing cataleptic trance on prisoners from a long range.

In reality, Esdaile demonstrates the magical properties of mesmerism first and thereafter claims to present scientific, irrefutable facts to validate mesmerism. But while publishing these mesmeric facts, he deliberately inverts the order. He begins like any other man of medicine seeking validation for a so-called pseudo-scientific mode of healing wishing to see it included in the pharmacopoeia. It is only towards the conclusion of this book that he reveals his real intention. He had been preparing his reading audience for being able to accept the so-called wondrous workings of mesmerism in which he seems to have believed more than anyone else. This revelation is surely a disappointment for the avid researcher who had by this time developed a supporting stance, albeit unawares, towards this unsung hero of alternative medical cure. The actual reason behind refusal to incorporate mesmerism into the annals of institutional medicine also becomes apparent. Institutional medicine based itself upon hard-core, verifiable evidences, not subjective proofs. After this realisation, the perhaps deliberate erasure of traces of evidence of mesmeric cure from the annals of colonial history of medicine hardly seems unfair.

REFERENCES

Esdaile, James. 1847. *Mesmerism in India and its Practical Application in Surgery and Medicine*. Hartford: Silas Andrus and Son.

Ernst, Waltraud. 2004. "Colonial Psychiatry, Magic and Religion. The case of Mesmerism in British India." *History of Psychiatry* 15(1):057-071.

In: Imperial Maladies
Editors: D. Bandyopadhyay et al.
ISBN: 978-1-53611-863-6

Chapter 9

KING'S DISEASE: TUBERCULOSIS IN COLONIAL CALCUTTA (1900-1947)

Suvankar Dey*
Department of History, Jadavpur University,
Kolkata, West Bengal

Colonial expansion not only brought exotic diseases to the colonies, but drastically changed their aetiologies. In the case of America, Europeans brought deadly viruses and bacteria, such as small pox, measles, typhus, cholera, for which Native Americans had no immunity as the native population had no previous contact with old world diseases, they were immunologically defenseless. It is estimated that 80% -90% of the Native American population was decimated within the first 100-150 years following the discovery of Columbus. (Nunn and Qian 2010, 163-168) As we already see that, tuberculosis was not a new disease in India but as a result of colonisation along with the urbanisation and industrialisation the physical and social environment of the country had changed. Initially

* Corresponding author: Department of History, Jadavpur University (Main Campus), 188 Raja S.C. Mallick Rd., Jadavpur, Kolkata, West Bengal, India. PIN – 700032, Email: suvankar.dey17@gmail.com.

tuberculosis was considered to be widespread in the urban areas. However, after 1900, tuberculosis had spread to the rural areas through the migrant populations. (Rao 2006, 457-485) These populations were mostly from laborers who had been migrated to the cities and towns in search of work. Those infected by the disease had no other option but to return to the countryside. Thus in this way, tuberculosis had spread in the rural areas. In the beginning of the 19th century India, it was generally believed that there was hardly any TB occurrence in India. By the middle of the 19th century, TB was thought to be common in some districts particularly among English troops, and in some areas it was thought to be common among natives as well, such as in the districts of Madras.

Growing urbanisation, gradual clearance of forests leading to climate changes, increase in habitation and brick constructions have made Calcutta what it is today. The geographical map of Calcutta has been constantly changing for ecological reasons of the riverine Bengal Delta. Calcutta (today's Kolkata) was situated on the east bank of the river Hooghly in the latitude 22' 23' 47 and longitude 88'23' 34E and was exactly 86.213 miles away from the sea or the Bay of Bengal in the 18th century. From the 19th century onwards the British view of disease in Calcutta had changed dramatically. The city came to be increasingly imagined as a hotbed of tropical diseases.

The Britishers had regarded the city as 'a dangerous arena' where precious English lives were lost. Thus, Ronald Martin in his "Notes on medical topography in Calcutta" (1837) referred to it as, 'disease arising from the deteriorating conditions in Calcutta and urgent need for medical institutions for the laboring poor'. Sir John Strachey had given us a decaying picture of Calcutta in late 19th century in his book *India* (1903). He wrote:

> ......Compare for instance, what Calcutta was when Lord Lawrence became viceroy in 1864 and what it is now. This city, the capital of British India, supplies and excellent type of what has been everywhere going on. The filth of the city used to root away in the midst of the population in pestilent ditches, or was thrown into Hooghly; there to float backwards and forwards with every change of tide. To nine-tenth of the

> inhabitants' clean water was unknown. They drank either the filthy water of the river, polluted with every conceivable abomination, or the still filthier contents of shallow tanks. The river, which was the main source of ordinary filth; it was the great graveyard of the city. I forgot how many thousand corpses were thrown into it from the Governments hospitals and jails, for these practices were not confined to the poor and ignorant; they were followed or allowed, as a matter of course, by the officers of the government and the municipality. I remember the sights which were seen in Calcutta in those days in the hospitals, and jails and markets, and slaughter houses, and public streets. The place was declared, in official reports written by myself in language which was not, and could not be, stronger than the truth required, to be hardly fit for civilized man to live in. There are now few cities in Europe with which many parts of Calcutta need fear comparison, and although in the poorer quarters there still much room for improvement…there is hardly a city in the world which has made greater progress. (Hunter 1908, 474)

However, quite a few sanitary developments occurred in Calcutta especially in the second half of the 19th century. In 1864, the first Health officer of Calcutta was appointed. His function was the supervision of surface conservancy and condition of roads. Inspectors of markets acted as his general assistants. There were also appointments of six registers of births and deaths. The Calcutta Corporation was reconstituted by the municipal acts and definite sanitary obligations were imposed by the Calcutta Municipal Act of 1923.

From the Second half of the 19th century, the subject of tuberculosis and its prevalence had been discussed widely. For example, the Bengal Branch of British Medical Association was established in 1863. In one of their meeting held in 1868 on January the issue of tuberculosis was discussed. In that meeting, Dr. Ewart discussed the comparative increase in the number of tuberculosis patients in the Calcutta Medical College. Gobindra Chandra Chatterjee, one of the speakers pointed out how tuberculosis in Calcutta gradually increasing day by day due to the climatic and habitual changes of the people. He was also blaming the construction of the houses made of bricks which obstructed the free circulation of air.

But however in general medical men of Bengal still believed that tuberculosis was rare in India and very few people were attacked by this disease compared to other European countries, as Binoybhusan Roy points out. (Roy 2005, 324-25) Soorjo Coomar Goodeve Chuckerbutty recorded that phthisis was rapidly fatal among the natives and East Indians and counted many victims annually. (Dasgupta and Bhattacharya 2014)

However, there was a great deal of paucity of statistics and sources regarding tuberculosis in Bengal in general and India in particular. Throughout the colonial period, deaths were reported by the ignorant village headmen or watchmen who describe every kind of illness as 'fever'. (Fox 1912, 294-98) Thus large proportion of cases of tuberculosis was hidden away under different headings. A.C. Ukil wrote in The Calcutta Municipal Gazette in an article

> We have reason to believe that the medical profession and public health officers have not yet co operated with the provisions of the law as they should have done in the interests of public health reform. The result is that a large proportion of tuberculosis cases is being wrongly entered under the heads of fever, respiratory disease and the various categories of infantile mortality from recent enquires made by us and other workers, it appears that nearly 50% of the deaths under other heads and that very few of infantile and higher age period deaths from tuberculosis are recognized and entered as such. (Ukil 1938)

The Public Health Commissioner in his annual report for the year of 1933 suggested that, a rough estimate of tuberculosis mortality might be made on the assumption that about 10-20% of the deaths under "fever" and about 20% of those under "respiratory disease" were actually due to pulmonary tuberculosis. Sir Leonard Rogers, I.M.S., examined 1000 fatal cases in the very feverish district of Dinajpur in lower Bengal in 1903. He remarks:

> .... I thus found that one third of the deaths attributed to fever were due to diseases such as dysentery, tumors, etc., in which fever was not even a marked symptom; another third were caused by such diseases such

> as pneumonia, bronchitis, phthisis (the last consisting 9% of total) and typhoid; while the remaining third were probably duo for the most part to malaria and kala azar…. (Lankester 1920, 21)

A very similar view had been shared by the Lieutenant C.J. Fox in a paper at the All India Sanitary conference held in Madras, 1912:

> …. I would not like to say India was not a civilized country, but in a matter of statistics we have not attained to any degree of reliability. As long as the registration of deaths is left to the village *chowkidar* in villages or registration clerk in towns, we can never hope for reliable statistics in regards to mortality in any disease, particularly in disease such as tuberculosis, deaths from which might quite easily be attributed to other conditions such as fever, bronchitis, pneumonia, diarrhoea, and dysentery. We have consequently to rely on statistics such as they are, for an idea of the mortality from this disease. The sanitary commissioners' reports contain figures showing mortality from this disease among troops and jail population, but there are no figures for the general population of India. But if the disease is so prevalent in countries like England, Ireland and America, with improve sanitation and less overcrowding, it is safe to assume that it is widely prevalent in India. (Fox 1912, 295)

Major General Sir John Megaw in 1933 estimated that there were probably two million cases of tuberculosis in India. His conclusion was: "tuberculosis is evidently very widespread throughout the villages of India but is specially serious in Bengal, Madras, the Punjab and Bihar and Orissa" (Megaw 1938, 623). In Bengal, there were some local surveys on tuberculosis in the first decade of the 20th century, which were carried out by Leonard Rogers (1904), Stewart and Proctor (1906-07), Bently (1911-12), these surveys, revealed that the disease was widely distributed in different parts of Bengal. In 1909, The Medical section Asiatic Society of the Bengal discussed the issue of tuberculosis and they adapted the following resolution:

> The medical section of the Asiatic society of Bengal having discussed the subject of tuberculosis disease in Bengal and its wide

> prevalence, are of the opinion that it is extremely common cause of great suffering and mortality, both among the European and Indian communities, and therefore venture to call the attention of the government of India and local government, to the urgent necessity for providing a properly equipped sanatorium for the treatment of early phthisis, such as has now been provided with the most satisfactory results in nearly all civilized countries. (Roy 1998, 76)

ALL INDIA SANITARY CONFERENCES AND THE QUESTION OF TUBERCULOSIS IN CALCUTTA

For the official point of view, it was not until the year 1911, that medical practitioners and sanitary officials believe in prevalence of tuberculosis in India. For the first time, the acknowledgement came from the medical professionals at their 'First All India sanitary conference (Bombay, 1911)'. The proceedings which were held in the council chamber of the Bombay secretariat, on November 13 and 14, 1911, opened with the following speech by the president:

> There still remain however, numerous sanitary research problems in India, as yet almost untouched. Some of these problems will I understand be brought before us by the provincial sanitary commissioners and deputy commissioners……….. in particular I may mention tuberculosis. Tuberculosis accounts for more than 75,000 deaths per annuam in the United Kingdom and the interesting report recently published by Dr. Turner, Health officer of Bombay, shows that the mortality from this disease in large cities like Bombay and Calcutta is already considerably higher than in Glasgow, Birmingham or Manchester[1].

In this conference, Kailash Chander Bose, LMS, in a paper titled "Spread of tuberculosis in Calcutta" pointed out the high prevalence of tuberculosis in Calcutta. With the help of the sanitary reports of the local

[1] The Proceedings of the first All India Sanitary Conference held at Bombay on the 13th and 14th November, 1911. p-2.

governments he showed how "tuberculosis is vigorously pushing its way through the crowded streets and lanes of the populous city of Calcutta and no step has yet been taken to resist its course". According to him:

> Within the last twenty years it has taken a firm hold on Calcutta from the rate at which it has been spreading it is no exaggeration to say that at no distant date it will be a very serious problem. The tool which Calcutta and its suburbs annually pay to the assessor of death on this head is simply appalling. (Bose 1911, 133)

He went on saying:

> We may grudge to pay a penny over the fixed municipal rates to the assessor of the corporation for carrying out certain important improvements, and we may move, heaven and earth to rescue us from the oppression, but we are offering no opposition to the demands of the ruthless assessor of tuberculosis. (Ibid, 137)

He mentioned that there was the lacuna of proper maintenance of the system of the registration of causes of death, but more or less about nearly one eighth of the total number of deaths in Calcutta was due to tuberculosis. He pointed out various leading causes including overcrowding, housing conditions, habits of spitting in the roads which in many ways helped to spread the disease. He had also suggested some remedies for eradication of this disease in Calcutta.

At The Second All India Sanitary Conference (Madras, 1912) there was an increasing discussion on tuberculosis. The need for an investigation into some of the problems connected with tuberculosis in India had been felt at the discussion on the subject at this conference:

> That statistics appear to show that this disease is rapidly increasing in India, especially in urban areas, but that it is doubtful whether the increase is real or apparent only and due to such causes as more accurate diagnosis and registration. In view of the importance of this question a full and thorough inquiry seems desirable….

In this conference, different views on anti tuberculosis program such as anti tuberculosis societies, establishment of sanatoria and dispensaries, improved ventilation of schools and homes, sanitation of towns and villages had been discussed. P.S. Chandrasekhar Professor of Bacteriology, Madras Medical College brought tuberculosis to the notice (Rao 2006, 459-483) of all medical practitioners as an important public health problem. He urged the conference to pay due attention to tuberculosis as it was 'fairly widespread' in the various parts of India.

Another interesting paper of this conference was, titled "Tuberculosis and its relation to public health" by Lieutenant C.J. Fox. The author presented his paper with the aim

> to draw attention not so much to what India is doing, as to what India might and should do for the eradication of this disease which, if the facts were appreciated, is more insidious and more to be dreaded than plague. (Fox op. cit, 294)

In the third All India sanitary conference (1914, Lucknow) Dr. Lankester strongly argued that situation of tuberculosis was horrible throughout India. He was also strongly believed in the value of tuberculin treatment. Soon he had been asked by the Indian Fund Research Association to carry out the investigation of tuberculosis in India.

REPORT BY ARTHUR LANKESTER ON TUBERCULOSIS WITH REFERENCE TO CALCUTTA

Dr. Arthur Lankester was the first person who had made detailed inquiry about the situation regarding tuberculosis in India. He travelled throughout India (including Burma). (Lankester 1920) During the eleven months of actual travelling (July 1914 to June 1916), covering a distance of nearly 35,000 miles, 85 cities were visited, including 29 out of the 30 which contained a population of over 100,000 inhabitants. He visited 9 native states during his tour across Hyderabad, Mysore, Gwalior, Indore,

Bhopal, Udaipur, Jaipur, Jodhpur, and Bharatpur. He spoke to many people obtaining information and advice from them. He had also visited many different institutions including hospitals, dispensaries, and sanatoriums.

The object of his inquiry had three major aims first, to obtain more exact knowledge than had hitherto been available about the actual prevalence of consumption in India; secondly, to investigate the causation of the disease with special reference to any points of difference or contrast as compared with what has been observed in other countries; and thirdly, to arrive at some definite conclusion as to what measures of prevention appeared to give the promise of an ultimate success. With regard to the prevalence of tuberculosis he came to the conclusion that in certain areas the prevalence of tuberculosis had certainly been increased. He mentioned, that lower Bengal was the most extreme region, where tuberculosis penetrated to a large extent. On his investigation of Calcutta, he said:

> The tuberculosis death rate here has remained almost stationary for many years past, the total deaths during 1919 being 1889, giving a death rate of 2.1 per mile. Here, however as in the case of Bombay and Madras, the incidence of the disease is concentrated on central and greatly overcrowded areas where the tuberculosis death rate probably rises to 4.0 or even higher. The extensive suburbs of the city are, comparatively speaking free from disease. In 1913 phthisis caused more deaths than either of the accurate infectious diseases, although both plague and cholera were present in an epidemic form. Taking into consideration the large number of people-students, laborers and others-who return to their homes at a distance after having, became infected with the disease in the city, it is impossible to avoid the conviction that the above figures fail to indicate the real mortality. Sir Leonard Rogers as a result of careful series of analysis of the post mortem Calcutta examinations made in connection with the Calcutta hospitals for a period of 22 years, found that no fewer than 17 per cent of the total deaths had been due to the tuberculosis disease, while in 25 per cent of the cases examined distinct signs of tuberculosis were found. (Ibid, 46)

Dr. Lankester made large number of recommendations in his investigation. He was possibly the first who realised tuberculosis the problem of the nation where significant money and time should be spent to conquer the menace. Thus, in 1915, the government of India circulated to all the presidencies a comprehensive report submitted by him on the prevalence of the tuberculosis along with certain suggestions. After the publication of this report in 1915, medical and sanitary officials had started to recognise that tuberculosis was widespread among general population in Bengal.

Prevalence of the Disease

Kailash Chander Bose, a Doctor by profession, in a paper read at the first All India Sanitary conference had provided an account of the death rate due to tuberculosis in Calcutta, during the time period: 1876-1891 (sixteen years)

Table 1. The spread of tuberculosis in Calcutta

YEAR	DEATH RATE
1876	407
1877	361
1878	302
1879	299
1880	454
1881	482
1882	482
1883	540
1884	525
1885	516
1886	536
1887	468
1888	572
1889	666
1890	743
1891	729

Source: *Kailash Chandra Bose, The spread of tuberculosis in Calcutta*, All India sanitary conference, Bombay 1911, p-134.

The author of this article informs us that with the advent of the new century, tuberculosis in its various forms was regularly progressing in Calcutta. He noted that, amongst the females in Ward no 14, Hindus in Ward no 4, Mohammedan females in Ward no 5, four had been badly suffering from tuberculosis. The men living in Ward no.4 were especially liable to diseases of the respiratory tract and phthisis alone carried off a good number of them (Bose 1911, 133-137). While in 1901, tuberculosis had accounted 1064 deaths in Calcutta, in 1904 the deaths from tuberculosis was increased by the 1608 deaths. He had given many reasons for the spread of the disease; some of the important factors were being overcrowding, town planning, the effect of urbanisation, etc. Kailash Chander clearly pointed out that:

> ....the disease has already spread all over the town and has not even spared in the quarters in which dwell the most intelligent and wealthy classes of its people". (ibid., 133-137)

H.M. Crake, Health officer of Calcutta has shown in his report for the year of 1921 that mortality figures from tuberculosis had been increasing. It had risen over 40% and one of Bengal's most urgently needed institution would be a tuberculosis sanatorium for the city of Calcutta, as quoted in The Indian Medical Gazette (May 1923, 233)[2]. In 1926, Dr. E. Muir in an article in Indian Medical Gazette stated that "while malaria is the most prevalent and perhaps fatal disease in the country district of Bengal, tuberculosis is undoubtedly the most fatal disease in larger towns". (Muir 1926, 326)Indian cities were inextricably associated with the disease of tuberculosis. The Table 2 below by Dr. Lankester shows that the mortality from tuberculosis had been generally high in three presidency cities:

[2] Quoted in *Indian Medical Gazette*, 1923, May, p -233.

Table 2. Statement Showing the Number of Deaths from Tuberculosis in Calcutta, Bombay and Madras, 1904-1919

YEAR	CALCUTTA		BOMBAY		MADRAS	
	DEATHS FROM TB	TB RATE PER MILE	DEATHS FROM TB	TB RATE PER MILE	DEATHS FROM TB	TB RATE PER MILE
1904	1608	1.8	3548	4.57	318	0.6
1905	2052	2.4	3183	4.10	832	1.6
1906	2201	2.6	4052	4.14	736	1.4
1907	2241	2.6	3440	3.51	641	1.2
1908	2101	2.5	3023	3.09	717	1.4
1909	1919	2.3	2862	2.92	774	1.4
1910	1971	2.3	2830	2.90	459	0.9
1911	2060	2.3	2694	2.75	760	1.5
1912	1931	2.3	2794	2.85	672	1.3
1913	2196	2.5	2452	2.19	481	0.9
1914	2137	2.4	1889	1.92	738	1.4
1915	1920	2.1	1710	1.74	759	1.5
1916	1738	1.9	1902	1.94	876	1.7
1917	1539	1.7	2118	2.16	1067	2.1
1918	1826	2.0	2513	2.56	1488	2.9
1919	1889	2.1	2780	2.83	1309	2.5

Source: *Arthur Lankester, Tuberculosis in India: its prevalence, causation and prevention*, Calcutta 1920, p-45.

Table 3. Deaths of Tuberculosis in Bengal Towns and Rural Areas (1921-1924)

YEAR	RURAL AREAS		TOWNS		TOTAL FOR BENGAL	
	DEATH	RATE PER MILE	DEATH	RATE PER MILE	DEATH	RATE PER MILE
1921	1394	0.03	2261	0.09	4055	0.01
1922	1496	0.03	2981	1.0	4477	0.01
1923	2079	0.04	2283	0.09	4492	0.01
1924	2326	0.05	3251	1.0	5577	0.01

Source: Taken from, Dr. E. Muir, Tuberculosis in Bengal, *Indian Medical Gazette*, 1926, July, P-326.

The reports of the Health officer of Calcutta show an average mortality during the years 1919 to 1923 of 2104 or about 3.3 per thousand of the population. (Ibid, 326) Sir Leonard Rogers provides us with figures from the post mortem records of the Medical College Hospital, Calcutta which show that 16.1% of the cases examined by him were due to phthisis. (Moller 1927, 332) From the reports of the Director of public health of Bengal, it was clear that, the disease appeared to be spreading from the towns and increasing in the rural areas (during the years 1921-1924 an average death rate of 0.95 per thousand in the towns and 0.037 per thousand in the rural areas). (Muir 1926, 326) There is a tendency of tuberculosis to spread from the towns to the villages. The following figures supplied by the Director of public health Bengal during the years 1921-1924 demonstrate the fact.

It is very interesting to note that most of the insurance companies operated their head offices from Calcutta and consequently the major portion of the work done in the peninsula referred to the city of Calcutta. Edward Houseman had shown in 1926, an excellent article of the death claims of the Indians as well as European on the major diseases. Interestingly enough, the Indian death claims of tuberculosis were quite higher than European counterparts.In his annual report for 1933, The Public Health Commissioner stated that

> Tuberculosis is now almost certainly one of the main public health problems in India, ranking probably next to malaria in this respect. In fact, it may be regarded as an epidemic disease. Bengal Public Health Report for the year of 1933 by Dr. R.B. Khambata noted that during this year deaths reported from phthisis numbered 14,802 in the province in 1933 showing an increase of 3001 against the previous year. The increase was shared to the extent of 2,583 by the rural areas and 418 by the towns, of which Calcutta was responsible for 315. The provincial death rate from phthisis showed an increase of 30.4%. The increase in the rural areas and towns was by 33.3 and 13.0%, respectively while that in Calcutta was by 14.2%, 70.6% of the phthisis deaths in all towns occurred in Calcutta alone. Eleven towns reported death rate above the provincial urban average (1.0). Pabna recorded the lowest rate (.04 per mile. In 1933,

Calcutta returned the highest death rate (2.17 per mile) from phthisis followed by Darjeeling (1.35)[3].

There were 11,130 deaths registered from phthisis in the rural districts and towns of the Bengal presidency during the year of 1933. (Ibid., 65-67)

Bengal Public Health Report gave detailed estimate of deaths from tuberculosis of the 24 Pargana District for the year 1933 where Calcutta had showed highest rate of mortality:

L.M. Biswas, Health officer of Calcutta had shown in his report of 1934 that mortality rate from tuberculosis in Calcutta was increasing year by year. He opined that, in 1934, almost whole of the mortality from tuberculosis was due to pulmonary tuberculosis. This variety of the disease accounted for 2759 deaths out of a total of 3053 deaths from tuberculosis or no less than 90% 294 deaths from other forms of TB were recorded in the year of the reported. He had noticed the high rate of mortality in the ward no 29(5.8p.m.), 24(3.8p.m), 19(3.8), 5(2.7p.m), 28(3.9p.m), 32(4.4p.m), 27(2.5p.m), 4(2.3p.m), 6(2.1p.m), 7(2.6p.m).[4]

According to him, the cases of tuberculosis in Calcutta might be briefly summarised as (1) poverty, under feeding, the struggle for existing under adverse conditions, etc. (2) ignorance and carelessness resulting sputum loaded with bacilli being expectorated all over the place (3) the *puradh* system of women (4) bad housing, a dark damp, ill ventilated hut in an open suburb was evidently just as deadly as badly lighted and ventilated room in the heart of the city. This report had also showed the high rate of mortality amongst young females between ages 15 and 30. It is important to note that, the death rates from tuberculosis in some of the important cities in India already exceeded the corresponding rates in well known cities abroad. The following figures are quoted from an editorial

[3] For details see, Bengal Public Health Report, For the year 1933 by Dr. R.B. Khambata, D.P.H., Director of Public Health, Bengal, Superintendent, government Printing press, Alipore, Bengal 1935.

[4] Report of health officer of Calcutta for the year 1934, by L.M. Biswas, L.R.C.S (Edin), D.T.M & H (camb), D.P.H (LOND,). P-28.

entitled "Tuberculosis as a public health problem in India" in the 1941 October issue of the *Indian Medical Gazette*[5]:

Table 4. Death claims of the Commercial Union Assurance and The Phoenix Assurance Company

DISEASE	INDIAN (%)	EUROPEAN (%)
Pneumonia	12.2	9.6
Heart Failure	7.9	15.9
Apoplexy	5.2	4.1
Phthisis	6.9	3
Diabetes (Including Carbuncle)	4.9	2.4
Liver Diseases (Including Abscess)	4.2	3.6
Kala Azar	0.09	0
Malarial Fever	2.8	0.6
Enteric Fever	4.2	3.9
Dysentary And Diarrhoea	5.1	2.7
Cancer	1.07	3.3

Source: *Medical aspects of life insurance in India, with special reference to Calcutta, Edward Houseman (*Chief medical officer in India to The Commercial union Assurance and The Phoenix Assurance Company), *Indian Medical Gazette*, June 1926, p-261

Table 5. Bengal Public Health Report for the year 1933 by Dr. B. R. Khambata

NAME OF DISTRICT AND TOWNS	PHTHISIS	
24 PARGANA DISTRICT	DEATHS	RATIO
South Sundarban	12	.3
Tollygunz	8	.2
Budge Budge	5	.7
Baranagar	28	.7
Kamarhati	20	.4
Rajpur	5	1.2
Baruipur	8	.6
Jaynagar	6	-
North Dum Dum	-	.4

[5] *Indian Medical Gazette*, Editorial, October, 1941, pp. 613-614

Table 5. (Continued)

NAME OF DISTRICT AND TOWNS	PHTHISIS	
	DEATHS	RATIO
24 PARGANA DISTRICT		
South Dum Dum	7	.2
Khardah	1	.2
Barackpur	4	.4
Panihati	5	.6
North Barakpur	10	-
Titagarh	-	.6
Garulia	8	.2
Naihati	-	-
Halisahar	5	.3
Kanchrapara	14	.2
Bhatpara	2	.2
Barasat	4	.9
Gobardanga	10	.5
Bashirhat	1	.1
Baduria	1	.1
Taki	-	-
Dum Dum	3	.1
Calcutta	2595	2.2

Source: *Bengal Public Health Report for the year 1933 by Dr. B.R. Khambata, D.P.H, Director of public health*, Bengal, superintendent, Government printing press, Alipore, Bengal 1935, p-200.

Table 6. Tuberculosis Deaths PEWR 100,000 Population

Paris	177	Crawnpore	432
Mexico	170	Lucknow	419
New York	128	Madras	290
Berlin	120	**Calcutta**	**230**
London	96	Bombay	140

Bengal was undoubtedly one of the worst suffers from tuberculosis. Tuberculosis was declared to be a noted disease on August 3, 1936, in municipal areas of Bengal, outside Calcutta. (Roy 1998, 76-80) Sir David Ezra, in the course of his presidential address at the 10th annual general meeting of the tuberculosis association of Bengal (held on March23, 1939) had opined that on a very modest computation, ten lakhs of people suffered from this disease and formed the force for the spread of infection. Tuberculosis alone killed one lakh of people in Bengal every year. After the famine of 1943, it is evidenced from Governmental publications and other non official observation that the serious problems posed by tuberculosis were manifold. To have an idea of the extent of morbidity and mortality from the disease, a survey was sanctioned by the Government of the two centers, one at Serampur and other at Barisal which were started in 1939. This survey had revealed a high incidence of infection and mortality from tuberculosis. At that time, series of anti tuberculosis measures were taken by the Government and other voluntary organisation for combating this scourge of mankind.

In the period under discussion, in colonial Calcutta, tuberculosis had been present everywhere. It was noted that the disease was contagious. Official and other non official writings in this period had confirmed that, the city of Kolkata was full of infected persons. 'Tubercular bacilli' the Invisible germs of tuberculosis had been present, not only in ill ventilated stuffy houses of the poor people but the disease had existed in the civilised section of the city. The situation was so horrible in that time, that someone could acquire this disease from an educational institution to a jute factory mill or from a restaurant to a cinema hall. The medical men at this time warned people not only to avoid congested areas but also to avoid many amenities of the colonial modernity. It was noted that, many aspect of colonial modernity (which in various way led to tuberculosis) had been repeatedly attacked and criticised by the indigenous medical practitioners. The disease was very high among women in *purdah*. The Health Officer of Calcutta highlighted these facts. Calcutta was inhabited by various communities of people. Each class were separate from the other, by their peculiar habits, customs, and mode of living. We have already discussed the living pattern of a Mohamedan housing condition of labour classes.

Tuberculosis had also been present in other sections of people. We have evidence to show that pulmonary tuberculosis had existed in Bengal Presidency Army, before 1900. Before 1941 no special facilities were provided in military hospitals for the treatment of soldiers suffering from tuberculosis. They were generally discharged from the armed force. Thus the policy of discharging military personnel suffering from tuberculosis before treatment was to a certain extent responsible for the dissemination of the disease in rural areas, particularly because the vast majority of personnel were recruited from such areas. (Raina and Prasad 1955, 525-529) Overcrowded military barracks, were bad in regard to ventilation, light and size[6]. In many barracks rooms, there was no air space, and sometime beds were so close that it was difficult and often impossible to walk between them. There was rapid growth of tuberculosis amongst children and students in India as well as in Bengal. The *Annual Report of the Medical Inspection of school children for the year 1933* revealed that there was sufficient number of school children in Bengal suffering from chest disease. Thus, total 183 schools were visited in 1933 by 41medical officers who were inspecting the health of 21,140 boys and 550 girls. About 414 or 1.44% of the students were suffering from bronchitis and other complication of the lungs[7]. It is interesting to note that, Rabindranath Tagore was enthusiastically in favour of open air education. His educational institutions like those in Santinikaton and Bolpur had been free from ill congested of dark four wall buildings. (Lankester 1920, 200)

The majority of people had been dying, untreated. A few cases were treated in medical college and other hospitals. The state of the Calcutta hospitals was a matter of shame. We find a horrible description of hospitals in Calcutta, 11 years even after the independence. Dr. B.P. Trivedi in his presidential address at the17th Bengal provincial medical conference in 1958 stated that:

> The condition is just like the third class passenger traffic of the old days. The whole existing set up is absolutely out of date for the present needs. Gone are the days when people would have to be persuaded, coaxed and cajoled to remove themselves to the hospitals. Now owing to

[6] The Imperial Gazetter of India, The Indian Empire, Vol. 1, Descriptive Portion, (Oxford: The Clarendon Press, 1909), pp. 521-526.

[7] 'Annual Report of the Medical inspection of school children for the year 1933' in Bengal Public Health Report for the year 1933 by Dr. R.B. Majumdar, (Alipore: Bengal Governtment Press, 1935), p. 85

> various factors, socio-economic and more hospital consciousness, people simply flock to the hospitals naturally. The load is tremendous to pieces. How can one expect the care and the treatment of the sick under this circumstance? The sick and suffering people are simply crowded together in beds on the floor space making it impossible even for the doctors, nurses and others to move in the wards.[8](Trivedi 1958, 301)

The growth of Calcutta as an industrial city with its negative effects, in many ways helped the spread of tuberculosis. Pollution from different sources had indirectly been responsible for the development of tuberculosis in human body. Wealthy people could afford the sanatorium treatment and sometimes they went to Madras and other south Indian states where sanatorium treatment made valuable progress. The poor, the most affected by the disease had no such option and hence, were helpless. Moreover, in colonial Calcutta, there was no proper registration of deaths due to this disease.

REFERENCES

Biswas, L. M. 1935. Report of health officer of Calcutta for the year 1934.

Bose, Kailash Chander. 1911. *The spread of tuberculosis in Calcutta* Appendix A to the proceedings of the First All India Sanitary Conference held at Bombay on 13th and 14th November, 133-137.

Dasgupta, Nupur. & Amit, Bhttachary. eds. 2014. *Essays in History of Science, Technology and Medicine.* Kolkata: Setu Prakashani.

Fox, C. J. 1912. "Tuberculosis and its relation to public Health", *Proceedings of All India Sanitary Conference*, November. Madras. 594-595.

Houseman, Edward. 1926. "Medical aspects of life insurance in India, with special reference to Calcutta". *Indian Medical Gazette*, June, 260-61.

Hunter, W. W. 1908. *The Imperial Gazetteer of India*, The Indian Empire, vol-*iv*, Adminstrative.

[8] Quoted in, *Journal of the Indian Medical Association*, Vol-31. No-4, August, 16, 1958, p. 301.

Khambata, R. B. 1935. *Public Health Report For the year 1933*. Alipore, Bengal: Government Printing Press, 65-67.

Lankester, Arthur. 1920. *Tuberculosis in India: its prevalence, causation and prevention*, Calcutta: Medical Publishers.

Majumdar, R. B. 1935. "Annual Report of the Medical inspection of school children for the year 1933". *Bengal Public Health Report for the year 1933.* Alipore: Bengal Government Press, 76-80.

Megaw, John. 1938. "Tuberculosis in India: A key problem." *The Asiatic Review*, Proceeding of the East India Association, October. 601-623.

Moller, C. Frimodt. 1927. "The Application of our knowledge of tuberculosis to Indian condition" *Indian Medical Gazette*, December. (Paper read at the 14th Indian science congress at Lahore, January, 1927).

Muir, E. 1926. "Tuberculosis in Bengal" *Indian Medical Gazette*, July.

Nunn, Nathan. & Nancy, Qian. (2010). "The Colombian Exchange: history of disease, food, and ideas" *The Journal of Economic Perspectives*, *29*, 2, 163-188.

Rao, B. Eswara. 2006. "From Rajayaks(h)ma (disease of kings) to Blackman's plague: perception on prevalence and aetiology of tuberculosis in the Madras Presidency, 1882-1947" *Indian Economic and social history Review*, 457-485.

Raina, B. L. & Bisheswar, Prasad. eds. 1955. *Official History of the Indian Armed forces in the Second World War 1939-1945: Medical services, medicine, surgery and pathology*. Combined Inter services Historical section India and Pakistan.

Roy, Binoy Bhusan. 2005. *Chikitsa Bijnaner Itihas* (In Bengali), Kolkata: Sahityalok.

Roy, Kabita. 1998. *History of public health colonial Bengal 1921-1947*, Calcutta: K P Bagchi & Company.

Trivedi, B. P. 1958. Presidential Address to the 17th Bengal provincial medical conference. (Quoted in *Journal of the Indian Medical Association*, August 16, 1958, 31. 4)

Ukil, A. C. 1938. 'Combating tuberculosis in Bengal: The outline of a scheme.' *Calcutta Municipal Gazette*, 9th April, 35-40.

Part 4.
Studies in Popular Fiction: Sensational Psychiatry

In: Imperial Maladies
Editors: D. Bandyopadhyay et al.
ISBN: 978-1-53611-863-6

Chapter 10

'WILDE DESIRE' ACROSS CULTURES: *DRACULA* AND ITS BENGALI ADAPTATIONS*

Prodosh Bhattacharya*† *and Abhirup Mascharak
Department of English, Jadavpur University, Kolkata, West Bengal

FROM SIN TO PATHOLOGY

> 'In modern western history, the category of the homosexual originates primarily from late-nineteenth-century notions, derived from medicine that defined same-sex desire as the product of disease, degeneracy, and moral inversion.' (Hertd 1998, 18)
>
> *Gilbert Herdt,*
> *Same Sex, Different Cultures: Gays and Lesbians across Cultures*

---

* Prefatory Note: The paper is a joint product. At the same time, it must be acknowledged that what had begun on my part as a general study of the two Bengali adaptations of Bram Stoker's *Dracula*, has been given its current focus and thrust by Mr. Abhirup Mascharak, who is pursuing doctoral research under me. *Prodosh Bhattacharya*

† Corresponding Author's address: Dept. of English, Jadavpur University Main Campus, 188, Raja Subodh Chandra Mallick Rd, Jadavpur, Kolkata, West Bengal 700032. Email: prodoshbhattacharya@gmail.com.

> 'The medical model of sexuality saw homosexuals not as sinners or criminals, but as abnormal individuals who were in need of a cure. Although some sexologists, including [Havelock] Ellis, saw homosexuality as inborn but not as a disease, much of sexual studies has been preoccupied with problematizing and investigating these "marginal" sexualities, and with thinking about how to "correct" the perceived pathologies …' (Mottier 2008, 39-40)
>
> *Veronique Mottier,*
> *Sexuality: A Very Short Introduction*

Discrimination against homosexuality definitely predates the nineteenth century, but, as the lines quoted above prove, this discrimination acquired a different hue in that era. Previously, 'deviant' sexuality was condemned on religious grounds. Those 'guilty' of it were called "sodomites" (after the Biblical tale of Sodom and Gomorrah, whose inhabitants were supposedly penalised for their 'deviance'), or, alternatively, "pederasts" (a term that was seen as belonging to a pre-Christian, and therefore, less moral, Europe). The increase in scientific studies, including those of the human mind and body, brought forth newer, though hardly more enlightened, notions about homosexuality, which was now seen as a disease. Speaking of this 'distinct semantic shift in the nineteenth century,' Sean Brady says that homosexuality now came to be regarded as 'a disorder of the emotions, instincts, and will caused by neurological or other organic problems' (Brady 2014, 45-46). One of the works which contributed enormously to this perception of homosexuality is Richard von Krafft-Ebing's *Psychopathia Sexualis* (1886).

The portrayal of homosexuality in Bram Stoker's *Dracula* (1897) has to be studied in the light of these newly-developed attitudes, though two specific incidents that took place in England in the years immediately before the publication of the book (and which Stoker was definitely witness to), also played a part in shaping his view of homosexuality. The first of these was the Cleveland Street Scandal, in which, it was suspected, multiple members of British Royalty and aristocracy had visited the brothel on the said street, where young male prostitutes provided services to the clients. The second was the much-publicised trial of Oscar Wilde, in which he was found 'guilty' of the charges of sodomy brought against him by the father of his lover, Lord Alfred Douglas. The realization that such distinguished members of British society could be homosexuals set off a frantic denunciation of homosexuality. The link between *Dracula* and these incidents has been noted by Talia Schaffer, who says:

> May 24, 1895 was a significant date for Stoker. On that date the English government convicted Oscar Wilde, and knighted Henry Irving and Stoker's brother Thornley … Dracula represents the ghoulishly inflated vision of Wilde produced by Wilde's prosecutors; the corrupting, evil, secretive, manipulative, magnetic devourer of innocent boys. (Schaffer 1997, 470-72)

In other words, *Dracula* was a paranoid response to the realisation that homosexuality is very much a part of English society, and Stoker's indictment of it is, as was the norm in the nineteenth century, coloured by medicality. A detailed study of the novel shall be undertaken in this paper to demonstrate as much. Before that, it is necessary to understand how the figure of Count Dracula has been queered in the novel.

The first instance where we get a hint of Dracula's queerness is in the memorable scene where he stops his three Brides from feasting on Harker. The Count, speaking '[i]n a voice which … seemed to cut through the air and then ring round the room', says:

> 'How dare you touch him, any of you? How dare you cast eyes on him when I had forbidden it? Back, I tell you all! This man belongs to me!' (Stoker (1897)1997, 43)[1]

The Norton editors tell us in a footnote that '[t]his proprietary sentence recurs over and over again in Stoker's working notes. The phrase *belongs to me* underlies *Dracula*'s vision of love, sexuality, nation, religion, and humanity itself' (Ibid., fn. 9).

---

[1] Bram Stoker, *Dracula* (first published in 1897), ed. Nina Auerbach and David J. Skal (New York: W.W. Norton and Company, 1997). We have used this edition throughout the paper.

Later, when Dracula comes to London, his depredations have been described by Christopher Craft as follows:

> [O]nce in England, Dracula, observing a decorous heterosexuality, vamps only women, in particular Lucy Westenra and Mina Harker. The novel, nonetheless, does not dismiss homoerotic desire and threat; rather it simply continues to diffuse and displace it. Late in the text, the Count himself announces a deflected homoeroticism when he admonishes [his opponents] thus: "My revenge is just begun! … Your girls that you all love are mine already; and *through them you and others shall yet be mine* … (… italics added) [267]. Here Dracula specifies the process of substitution by which "the girls that you all love" mediate and displace a more direct communion among males. (Craft 1997, 446-48)

The phrase 'through them you and others shall yet be mine' offers a hint about how Stoker viewed homosexuality. The one thing people fear most about any disease is its spread. That is the reason that those suffering from leprosy were once banished to colonies outside human settlements (in some parts of the world, this is still the practice), or why those diagnosed with the HIV were seen as fit to be locked away. Whether or not the disease is contagious, the fear of contracting it has often led to discriminatory practices against the patients. Ever since homosexuality came to be regarded as pathology, the fear of homosexuals 'turning' other people into diseased individuals like themselves also grew prevalent. Despite all the progress made by the gay rights movement throughout the twentieth century and thereafter, this idea that homosexuals spread their sexual inclinations among others continues to hold currency across the world and used by politicians and policy-makers to pass discriminatory provisions against the LGBT community. In 1978, the Briggs Initiative, aimed at preventing gays and lesbians from working in California's public schools, was undertaken on the grounds that 'the advocating, soliciting, imposing, encouraging or promoting of private or public homosexual activity' would 'adversely affect students or other employees'. John Briggs, the creator of the aforementioned Initiative, warned, "Homosexuals want your children … They don't have any children of their own. If they don't recruit children or very young people, they'd all die away. They don't have any means of replenishing." Years later, in 2013, Russia passed a similar, federal law—popularly referred to as the Gay Propaganda Law in the English-speaking media—which forbids any mention or discussions about homosexuality in the presence of minors. As with the Briggs Initiative, this too has been done, as Vladimir Putin puts it, to "protect the children." The necessity to safeguard the young from any sort of exposure to homosexuality has been further clarified by the politician Vitaly Milonov, who says, "Gay propaganda can influence children. Look at Germany, where statistics indicate that 12 percent of the population is gay. Statistics also show that 40 percent of men in Berlin have tried homosexual sex. This cannot be explained by biology." Briggs, Putin and Milonov are all driven by the concern that children, if placed in proximity to homosexuals or told that they are normal, would become gay themselves, and that this is what the homosexuals want, for they, as Briggs said, "don't have any means of replenishing." In non-western countries, there is often an added layer to the homophobia: homosexuality is described there as something imported from the west, a corrupting influence against which indigenous cultures must guard themselves. Robert Mugabe's statement that homosexuality is a "white disease", or the former Indian Health Minister Ghulam Nabi Azad's remark that "the disease of Men having Sex with Men (MSM), which was found more in the developed world, has now unfortunately come to our country", and that this supposed ailment is "fast spreading", propagate the disease model of homosexuality by 'Other-ing' non-heterosexual orientations as fundamentally white, western afflictions. Non-whites are urged to stay away from western values if they do not want to be infected with such perversion. In all of these instances, the common, unifying factor is the belief that homosexuality is not innate but learned, and Dracula's remark that all the men shall 'yet be mine' is but an expression of this very school of thought: that he shall, via the women he has already seduced, extend his control to the males, who are his actual targets and who he shall queer accordingly. Dracula and his Brides, being undead, cannot reproduce, so the only way they can increase their tribe is by force and seduction, which is what they do. The bite on the neck, then, is an act of penetration that stands for sexual violation, and the subsequent transformations in the victims are the manifestation of the queerness they have been infected with.

Against this queer antagonist, Stoker pits the 'Crew of Light' – led by Abraham Van Helsing, and assisted by Jonathan Harker, John Seward, Arthur Holmwood, and Quincey Morris. Stoker, throughout the novel, is at pains to remind his readers of the collective heterosexuality of this group. Van Helsing's wife, though "no wits, all gone" (Stoker 1997, 158), is alive; Jonathan is engaged to Mina Harker; and Seward, Holmwood, and Morris are suitors of Lucy. During a conversation the men have about donating blood to the ailing Lucy Westenra, Van Helsing says, in response to Seward's statement that Holmwood's donating blood to Lucy had made her his bride, "If so that, then what about the others? Ho, ho! Then this so sweet maid is a polyandrist, and me, with my poor wife dead to me, but alive by Church's law … am bigamist." (Ibid.) By describing the donation of blood to a woman in the terms of matrimony and sexual intercourse, the novel embeds all these men in a heterosexual matrix. That Stoker associates this all-round heterosexuality with healthiness – literally – is proved by the profession he assigns to Van Helsing, the leader of the Crew: he is a distinguished member of the medical fraternity, and so is his aide Seward. If vampirism is the 'disease' that Dracula is spreading in London, and if he is (as already evinced) a Wilde-inspired queer figure, then his vampirism is a metaphor for homosexuality, and when the Crew of Light led by a doctor, and comprising another doctor, kills the Brides of Dracula[2] and the Count, they are eliminating the 'threat' of homosexuality to make the society, so to speak, 'healthier.' Even before that, we see Van Helsing treating Lucy, after she is infected by Dracula, both by surrounding her

[2] The three brides do target the male Jonathan Harker at the beginning of the novel (on which more later), but towards the end, they also attempt a very same-sex seduction of Mina:

> Then, alas! … the wheeling figures of mist and snow came closer, but keeping ever without the Holy circle. Then they began to materialize, till … there were before me in actual flesh the same three women that Jonathan saw in the room, when they would have kissed his throat … They smiled ever at poor dear Madam Mina; and … they twined their arms and pointed to her, and said in those so sweet tingling tones …'Come, sister. Come to us. Come! Come!' (Stoker, *Dracula*, Norton Critical Edition), 317.

with garlic flowers and crucifixes, and by providing her with four blood-transfusions. This strange mix of religious rituals and medical procedures is reflective of the homophobia of the era, which was both informed by the puritanical religious thoughts of the preceding centuries while simultaneously influenced by the recently developed medical model that looked upon such 'deviance' as something to be tackled by doctors rather than priests.

A further portrayal of homosexuality as disease comes in the form of Renfield. An inmate of Seward's lunatic asylum, we do not know what he is there for, but his devotion to Dracula, even though Renfield has not been vampirised, indicates that he may well have been imprisoned for reasons pertaining to sexual deviance. He certainly addresses the Count in terms that are tinged with homoeroticism. 'The bride-maidens,' he tells Dr Seward, 'rejoice the eyes that wait the coming of the bride; but when the bride draweth nigh, then the maidens shine not to the eyes that are filled' (Stoker 96-97). The Norton editors explain this 'biblical-sounding rhapsody' as equating 'Dracula's advent with the coming of the Messiah,' but go on to point out that '[t]he New Testament never refers to Jesus as a bride, though he is occasionally a bridegroom.' However, they add, that in Revelation 21.2, New Jerusalem is described as '"coming down from God out of heaven, prepared as a bride adorned for her husband."' (Ibid., 97, fn. 1) Renfield may, as the editors say, 'exalt not so much the coming of Dracula as the glorious new dispensation Dracula promises,' (Ibid.) but the homoeroticism is undeniable. When he first escapes from Seward's asylum to the deserted house bought by Dracula, this is how he is found talking to the latter's unseen presence by his captors:

> 'I am here to do your bidding, Master. I am your slave, and you will reward me, for I shall be faithful. I have worshipped you long and afar off. Now that you are near, I await your commands, and you will not pass me by, will you, dear Master, in your distribution of good things?' (Stoker 1997, 98)[3]

[3] Stoker, *Dracula*, Norton Critical Edition, 98. As the editors point out (98, fn.3), Dracula is a blasphemous parody of Jesus in that he feeds his followers by transforming blood into life, as

Later, his attempts to leave his "Master" results in his death at the hands of Dracula. To Stoker, then, homosexuality is not only an illness, but an incurable one: those carrying it have to die in one way or the other to ensure the well-being of society at large; hence, the deaths of Dracula, his Brides, Lucy, and Renfield.

THREE FILM VERSIONS OF *DRACULA*: THE DISEASE MOTIF PERPETUATED

The homosexuality-as-disease motif, though subtextual, was palpable enough to be picked up by filmmakers across the world while adapting the novel to screen. In F.W. Murnau's *Nosferatu* (1922), Count Orlok's arrival in Bremen leads to an outbreak of plague, which ends only when he is killed. Before that, Orlok had been introduced as somebody who lives alone in his Transylvanian castle. Significantly, there are no Brides around. When Hutter (the Jonathan Harker counterpart) visits Orlok, he is greeted with a gleeful welcome ("I have waited long, so long, for you…"), and later, in a most suggestive scene, Orlok grabs hold of Hutter's bleeding finger and sucks on it greedily. A horrified Hutter stumbles backward, but the Count keeps cornering him, until Hutter is almost pushed into an armchair by the fireplace, and awakens next morning in a semi-supine position, with two bite marks on his throat. That night, the Count comes to Hutter again, this time in the young man's bedroom, with his shadow looming over and almost engulfing Hutter. These scenes—with Hutter cowering and trembling before the Count while the latter mercilessly bears down on him—are filmed like rape scenes, and thus lend a sexual dimension to the vampire's feeding on his victim. Orlok is not the only one responsible for Hutter's suffering, though. It is Renfield, re-named Knock here, who practically delivers Hutter into Orlok's hands by sending Hutter to Transylvania to negotiate the purchase of a house. Knock is well aware

---

Jesus did by transforming 'a handful of loaves and fishes into food for "four thousand men, beside women and children"'. (Matthew 15:23)

of what shall happen to Hutter once he reaches Orlok's castle: "The Count is rich, and free with his money. You will have a marvellous journey. And, young as you are, what matter if it costs you some pain—or even a little blood?" he says, leering at his young employee. An intertitle informs us that there are "many dark rumours about Knock", and his collusion with Orlok provides indications aplenty of what those rumours may be: what we have here is an intra-continental partnership between two disreputable, repugnant queer men, one of whom supplies the other with unsuspecting young male victims such as Hutter. Therefore, when one of these men comes to Bremen and brings the pestilence with him, and the other (Knock) is captured and placed in a psychiatric ward, a direct continuum is established between queerness, sexual perversion, and disease. Unsurprisingly, what rescues the world from the sexual pathology of the likes of Orlok and Knock is heterosexual love. Ellen, the devoted wife of Hutter, sacrifices her life to kill Orlok, in the process avenging what was done to her spouse and lifting the pall of plague from the city.

At least Murnau does not show Orlok transmitting vampirism through his bites, which Tod Browning's *Dracula* (1931), on the other hand, is only too glad to emphasise. Browning replaces Harker with Renfield in the first half of the film, as we see the latter go to the Count's castle, get vamped, and turn into a raving, crazy devotee of Dracula, with a thirst for blood, albeit the blood of small animals rather than humans.[4] Upon returning to England (with the Count in tow), Renfield is diagnosed as sick and put in Seward's sanatorium, where he keeps speaking of his "Master", who in fact uses Renfield's devotion to him to enter the sanatorium and get access to other victims, including Mina, who, in this film, is Seward's daughter. The fact that his liaison with Dracula has made Renfield 'sick', that a prominent symptom of this 'sickness' is the yearning for another man, and that the scene of him being vamped was concealed with a black fadeout, only heighten the associations between illness and homosexuality. This 'male-to-male blood ritual', as David Skal put it, was so obviously a 'homoerotic rite of passage' (Skal 2004, 97-98), that it could not possibly

[4] Van Helsing, though, apprehensively hints in one scene that Renfield's thirst for animal blood may culminate eventually into a desire for human blood.

have been put on the screen, because of Hays Code, which probably also explains the directive from the producer, Carl Laemmle Jr., that Dracula should 'go only for women and not men' (Towlson 2016, 43). The film also borrows from the disease motif in *Nosferatu* by having Renfield crave the blood of rats, which remind us of the plague in Murnau's film, and further link men like Renfield (and Dracula, whose eyes are described as red, like those of the rats) to disease-carriers.

Terence Fisher's *Dracula* (1958) refers to both *Nosferatu* by shifting much of the action to Germany, and Browning's film by using the blackout in the scene where the Count vamps Harker. The later seductions of Lucy and Mina, though, are clearly shown. These contrasting approaches make it clear that while the Count is a danger to all, what he does to men constitutes the bigger taboo.

One may note that in all the three films we see the Harker figure being actually preyed on, though this does not happen in the book, and Renfield, a secondary character in Stoker, is given far more importance in both Browning's film and Murnau's. Since Renfield, alongside Dracula, was the most clearly diseased figure in the novel, these additional bits in the films heighten the homophobia, which means that these adaptations, for all their deviations from their source material, are ultimately unable to escape the idea of homosexuality as pathology.

Hemendra Kumar Roy's Bengali Adaptation

It is this view of homosexuality that undergoes a noticeable change in *Bishalgarh-er Duhshasan* (*The Tyrant of Bishalgarh*, 1949), one of the most well-known Bengali adaptations of *Dracula*. The author, Hemendra Kumar Roy, includes the following, curious statement in his foreword to the novel:

> ... nowhere have I forgotten that *Dracula* is an outdated novel and my readers are ultra-modern(Roy 1949, rpt. 1964, foreword)[5]

Since Roy does not clarify what he means by 'outdated', it leaves room for speculation, and given the changes he made in his adaptation, which will soon be discussed, it is possible that he was referring to the very homophobia that marks much of Stoker's book. This interpretation gains more credence in the light of the fact that Roy's fiction, both for adults and children, is characterised by a distinct degree of homoeroticism that manifests itself in the most heroic and sympathetic of his characters, rather than the villainous or the comic ones. In *Aaleyar Aalo* (*The Elusive Illumination*, 1918), for instance, there is a prolonged scene of physical affection between a young widow and an older, married woman, and a much later work, *Priya O Priyo* (*The [Female] Beloved and the [Male] Lover*), features a homosexual couple, one half of whom, Piru Thakur, is created as an outcast hero who stands up to injustice when he sees it taking place. Roy's works for younger readers similarly has characters like Bimal and Kumar, the adventurer duo whose refusal to marry, articulated eloquently in *Kuber Purir Rahasya* (*The Mystery of the Palace of Riches*), coupled with the intimacy they share (which is expressed, variously, in books like *Himalaye-r Bhayankar* [*The Terror of the Himalayas*] and *Jerinar Kanthahar* [*The Necklace of the Czarina*]), hint amply at the actual tenor of their relationship. Even more pronounced is the relationship between Barun, a Robin Hood-like figure who loots the rich under the moniker 'Dinabandhu' (the friend of the poor), and his companion Arun, a writer: as traced over five novels,[6] it is, for all practical purposes, a romance, which takes on the hue of conjugality when they finally leave India to escape the law and go and settle in the forests of Borneo.

---

[5] Hemendra Kumar Roy, *Bishalgarh-er Duhshasan* (Kolkata: Abhyuday Prakash Mandir, 1949; rpt. 1964), foreword. This foreword is found only in this edition of the novel. It occurs on the leaf after the title page, facing the one giving publication details.

[6] Chronologically, these five novels are *Mayamriger Mrigaya* (*Hunting the Elusive*), *Bajra Aar Bhumikampa* (*Calamitous Times*), *Neelpatrer Raktalekha* (*Blood-Message of the Blue Letters*), *Byadher Phaand* (*The Hunter's Trap*) and *Suryakarer Dweep-e* (*In the Island of the Sun*).

In *Bishalgarh-er Duhshasan*, Roy similarly takes a more nuanced and positive view of homosexuality than Stoker did. On the one hand, the queerness in the Dracula figure (called Raja Rudrapratap Singha here) is both exacerbated and complicated, while on the other hand, the counterparts of Van Helsing and Jonathan Harker (Abinash-babu and Binoy Bhushan Bhowmick respectively) are much less manifestly heterosexual: indeed, their relationship is subtly queered in the novel. Roy was aided largely by the fact that he was writing his novel for an adolescent readership. An unwritten rule in children's literature is that sex must not figure in the writings, at least not too overtly, even in its heterosexual avatar. Indeed, it *is* the heterosexual avatar that people refer to when declaring the "no sex" rule, for it is assumed that homosexuality is, obviously, even more of a taboo topic to be broached in books written for children. Dracula's seduction of Lucy and Mina has unmistakable sexual undercurrents, so it must have been deemed 'proper' on the part of Roy when he removed both of these characters from *Bishalgarh-er Duhshasan*. This inevitably means, though, that Binoy, the Harker-figure, has no fiancée, and since there is no Lucy, there are no suitors for her either. The task of fighting Rudrapratap falls entirely to Binoy and Abinash-babu, the latter an unmarried man whose bachelorhood is insistently described at the beginning of the second part of the novel. This insistence reminds us of the similar vehemence with which Bimal and Kumar refuse to enter wedlock in *Kuber Purir Rahasya*. They do not want to marry because they see themselves as soul-mates: as Kumar puts it, "We eat, sleep, and travel together, and wish to die together too, so our opinions [in this case, about marriage] are also identical." (Roy 2005, 145. Translation ours) Abinash-babu does not have a companion yet when his bachelorhood is being described, but since his determination to not marry echoes Bimal and Kumar's, it is possible to interpret his outlook in a queer light as well. Indeed, once he meets Binoy, their relationship takes on a distinct erastes-eromenos dynamic. Before discussing that, though, it is necessary to see what Roy has done with Rudrapratap.[7]

[7] *Rudra* translates as 'terrible' and *Pratap* as 'might' or 'power'. The surname *Singha*, meaning 'lion', is a common title all over north India. The name therefore has connotations of the

Like Dracula, Rudrapratap lives in a castle with three Brides, and imprisons Binoy when the latter visits the castle. In the scene where Rudrapratap stops his Brides from feeding on Binoy, he thunders, "No one has any right over this man apart from me!" (Roy 1964, 25. Translation ours) Later, while restraining the Brides outside Binoy's room, Roy's Rudrapratap, most interestingly, utters in Bengali the sentence Stoker omitted from the British edition, "*Tonight is mine.* Your night will come tomorrow." (Ibid., 35. Translation ours, emphasis added)[8]. The addition of this line only underscores Rudrapratap's queerness vis-à-vis Dracula's. Once Rudrapratap arrives in Kolkata, he comes and perches on a tree outside Binoy's house every evening, and fixes his eyes – which Binoy recognizes as the Raja's – on Binoy's face. Add to this the fact that, in Kolkata, all of Rudrapratap's victims are male. One victim, Pulinbihari, the attack on whom is described in a newspaper report, is in his bed when Rudrapratap, in bat shape, lies on top of him, sucking his blood, until disturbed by the terrified cry of the victim's wife. This scene is remarkably similar to Carmilla/Mircalla's attack on Bertha in Le Fanu's novella *Carmilla*, a work itself noted for its queer undertones.

These facts may make it seem that Roy is even more intent than Stoker on associating homosexuality with vampirism, and using the latter as a metaphor for a disease that is being spread by the queer villain. The possibility of such a reading is undercut by the fact that, unlike those of Dracula, the victims of Rudrapratap die rather than turn into vampires themselves. Dracula is threatening because he can turn others into queer

fearsome and the predatory. The name of the kingdom is a compound of *Bishal*, 'massive' and *garh*, 'fortress', the latter corresponding to the Latin *castra*, 'fortified camps', which became the place-name element *chester/caster* in English.

[8] Dracula's words are quoted below as they appear in the 1899 American, rather than the 1897 British, edition:

> 'Back, back, to your own place! Your time is not yet come. Wait. Have patience. *Tonight is mine*. Tomorrow night, tomorrow night, is yours!' (52; emphasis mine, words added from fn. 2 on that page in Stoker, *Dracula*, Norton Critical Edition)

As the Norton editors say in their footnote to this speech, where they provide the sentence missing from the British edition, this is a bold statement 'that Dracula plans to feed on Jonathan. Stoker's deletion of the sentence was understandable, for it leads to a different novel, one probably unpublishable in 1897 England; Stoker may have imagined that the America that produced his hero Walt Whitman would be more tolerant of men feeding on men.' (Stoker, *Dracula*, Norton Critical Edition), 52, fn. 2.

beings like himself, but Rudrapratap does nothing of the sort, his own queerness notwithstanding. He does not 'spread' vampirism/queerness, thereby lessening the possibility of reading queerness as a contagious disease, and challenging the very notion that sexual orientation is something transmitted (like a disease) rather than being something innate. Therefore, the associations between homosexuality and pathology are far less pronounced as far as Rudrapratap is concerned. Moreover, unlike Dracula, he makes no grandstanding statements about taking over the human race and making them all "mine", which goes with the aforementioned fact that his victims do not become vampires. Rudrapratap, at worst, is like the wolves he commands: an animal on the hunt rather than a perversion intent on spreading itself like a plague. Furthermore, Abinash-babu is not a doctor, so the queerness-versus-medicine underpinnings of the antagonism between Van Helsing and Dracula are largely absent from the fight between Abinash-babu and Rudrapratap. Most importantly, Renfield is eliminated altogether from Roy's novel, leaving even less of a possibility for queerness to be read as a disease.

The queerness in Abinash-babu and Binoy is less evident, because Roy did not have for them a queer model as he did for Rudrapratap in the form of Dracula. It is revealing, nonetheless, that the relationship between them has more of the mentor-disciple tenor than does that between Van Helsing and his young companions. Binoy describes Abinash-babu as "Bengal's best occultist" (Roy 2005, 41, translation ours), thus putting the latter on a venerable position, to whom Binoy has come to seek aid in ridding the city of Rudrapratap. As the novel progresses, we see Binoy learning, step by step, about fighting vampires from Abinash-babu. First, he is instructed to wear, at all times, the sacred amulet he was given by the old innkeeper woman at Bishalgarh, for it is a definite safeguard against Rudrapratap. Abinash-babu demonstrates as much by making Binoy dangle this amulet in front of the vampire, who flees immediately. Later, in the mansion Rudrapratap has rented in Kolkata, Binoy and Abinash-babu are cornered by the vampire king, and while Binoy is paralyzed with fear as a result, Abinash-babu guides him to overcome his terror and flash the amulet at Rudrapratap again, which stops him in his tracks and makes him run for his life. After they have followed Rudrapratap to Bishalgarh, it is Abinash-babu who, at night, draws an enchanted circle and strictly instructs Binoy to stay within it to avoid any vampire attacks, and later, it is he who leads the charge against both the three Brides, and Rudrapratap.

The attempted seduction of Binoy by the Brides while he is sitting inside the circle deserves analysis in this regard. In *Dracula*, this seduction was done to lure Mina, and Van Helsing describes her response thus: "…my heart with gladness leapt like flame; for oh! the terror in her sweet eyes, the repulsion, the horror, told a story to my heart that was all of hope. God be thanked she was not, yet, of them" (Stoker 1997, 317). The seduction by three people of the same sex as her leaves Mina scared and dismayed rather than allured, and this gladdens Van Helsing in one more instance of Stoker's disapproving stance on homosexuality. In *Bishalgarh-er Duhshasan*, on the other hand, this seduction turns heterosexual when the Brides try it on Binoy. The words Binoy uses to account for his state of mind are notable: "I stood up and proceeded towards them like a swaying drunkard", "the world seemed to have stopped making any sense to me", "without knowing what I was doing, I took off my amulet" (Roy 2005, 61). These images of intoxication, confusion and lethal hypnotism are thus associated with heterosexual lure, and Binoy is prevented from giving in to it by his male companion, Abinash-babu, who grabs him by the arm at the right time and draws him back into the circle. Unlike Van Helsing, whose heterosexual-paternal influence, it is indicated, acts as a safeguard against the seduction of Mina by the Brides, Abinash-babu prevents his male apprentice from being lured by the opposite rather than the same sex. This is followed by his admonition of Binoy, at the end of which Binoy swears to Abinash-babu that he shall not "go astray" again. The specific Bengali word Binoy uses is *"pathachyuta"* (Ibid., 62). *"Pathachyuta"* and *"padaskhalan"* are related words, which literally mean 'going astray' and 'to slip', thus indicating a kind of lapse, but are used, normally, to denote a *sexual* lapse (or at least, what society mostly deems a sexual lapse). Binoy's use of this term to denote his almost-succumbing to the three Brides is significant. The Brides' beckoning of Binoy definitely had sexual undertones, and his regretful mention of his response, similar to the 'terror' and 'repulsion' felt by Mina towards the Brides, transfers the regret, the fear and the repulsion from same sex to opposite sex seduction. That it is the intervention of Binoy's same sex companion and mentor that stops the young man from crossing the circle imparts a distinct queerness to their relationship. As mentioned before, Binoy and Abinash-babu's camaraderie resembles the erastes-and-eromenos dynamic. 'According to the paradigm', says John F. Makowski, 'the older man, the *erastes*, partners with a younger man, the *eromenos* or *paidika*, in a relationship marked by asymmetry in that the *erastes*, being more mature, is something of a mentor to the younger and serves as role model and teacher of civic and military virtue…The chief hallmark of the *eromenos* is the physical beauty of youth along with the desire for the edification that association with the *erastes* will bring' (Makowski 2014, 491). Such a relationship was called pederasty, which Makowski sums up as 'homoerotic love in its conventional ancient form', 'whereby an older male loves a younger one' (Ibid., 490). This description is applicable almost in its entirety to Abinash-babu and Binoy's relationship. The asymmetry is obvious in the constant guidance Binoy needs in his fight against Rudrapratap from Abinash-babu, with instructions to fight vampires taking on both military (since it involves combat; in the end, there is even a fight and shootout between Binoy and Abinash-babu on the one hand and the gypsies who serve Rudrapratap on the other) and civic (because Rudrapratap's presence is a threat to the entire populace of Kolkata) significance. Binoy's physical beauty is mentioned, if only in passing, by the Brides during their seduction of him (Roy 2005, 61), and edification comes in plenty for Binoy in his conversation with Abinash-babu, most notably after the said seduction scene. Finally, there is the age gap between them—Abinash-babu is in his fifties while Binoy is much younger, as is the case in any erastes-eromenos relationship.

The differences in the sexual feelings of the characters in *Dracula* and *Bishalgarh-er Duhshasan* are perhaps clearest in the scene in both the books where the three Brides are killed. In Stoker, Van Helsing is extremely hesitant about carrying out the executions, and his hesitation is rooted in the sexual attraction he feels towards the Brides:

> She lay in her Vampire sleep, so full of life and voluptuous beauty that I shudder as though I have come to do murder … There is some fascination, surely, when I am moved by the mere presence of such an one, even lying as she lay in a tomb fretted with age and heavy with the dust of centuries … Yes, I was moved – I, Van Helsing, with all my purpose and with my motive for hate – I was moved to a yearning for delay … She was so fair to look on, so radiantly beautiful, so exquisitely voluptuous, that the very instinct of man in me, which calls some of my sex to love and to protect one of hers, made my head whirl with new emotion. (Stoker 1997, 319-20)

This may be contrasted with the unwavering grit of Abinash-babu as he finishes off the Brides, unperturbed by any of the feelings that held Van Helsing back. It is Binoy who feels a sense of foreboding and reservation about killing them, because, like Van Helsing, he thinks that the sleeping Brides look incredibly alive, and therefore, beheading them somehow tantamounts to murder. Unlike the Doctor, though, Binoy feels little in terms of sexual attraction to the Brides. His dilemma is more ethical than sexual. He takes note of their beauty, but this is preceded by his description of them as 'terrible-beauties', and later, he speaks of the 'ferocious disposition that is concealed beneath their outward appeal' (Roy 2005, 64). Van Helsing, too, is aware of the Brides' ferocious disposition, but even this awareness is coloured by thoughts of 'the beautiful eyes of the fair woman' opening and her 'voluptuous mouth' planting a kiss on the lips of the man who has come to kill her (Stoker 1997, 319). It may be instructive, in this context, to also recall that the very first meeting between Binoy and the Brides was bereft of any of the sexual arousal experienced by Harker. The latter, for all his fear, also speaks of his 'wicked, burning desire that [the Brides] would kiss me with those red lips' (Ibid., 42). He, even adds, 'It is not good to note this down, lest some day it should meet Mina's eyes and cause her pain: but it is the truth', and the bite from the first Bride is awaited 'in an agony of delightful anticipation' (Ibid.). None of this is felt by Binoy, who is only paralysed with fear (Roy 2005, 25). In other words, neither of Roy's heroes betray the sexual attraction that Van Helsing and Harker shake off only with a lot of difficulty, which further hints at the very different conceptualisation of Roy's characters as far as their sexuality is concerned.

It may be useful to look at Stoker's and Roy's differing views on homosexuality in conjunction with their political views. Stoker, a staunch believer in the British Empire, thought it beneficial for his native Ireland to remain a part of it. Unsurprisingly, then, the conflict between the protagonists and the antagonist in his most famous work has echoes of the colonial rivalries that Europe was witness to during the time. The Count's East European ancestry links him to Russia, and this link is highlighted when he travels from Transylvania to England on a Russian ship called the *Demeter* (Stoker 1997, 79). Relations between Britain and Russia had been strained throughout the nineteenth century, largely owing to what has come to be known as the Eastern Question. It began when the defeat of Turkey in the Russo-Turkish War of 1774 caused the Ottoman Empire to weaken, prompting the European powers, including the British and the Russians, to get involved in a power struggle to secure their commercial and military interests in the Ottoman-ruled regions, and also to step into the power vacuum created by the gradually disintegrating Ottoman regime. The resultant friction led to the Crimean War of the 1853. The parallel contest of the Great Game, or the rivalry between Britain and Russia to gain supremacy in Afghanistan, was also underway. It was only in 1895, a mere two years before the publication of *Dracula*, that the complication of the Great Game was believed to have been resolved. The anxiety of these rivalries has found their way into the novel. The arrival of the foreign Count on a Russian vessel, and his rapid vampirisation of multiple English citizens may well be read as an invasion of Britain by a rival power it has long been on hostile terms with, and the death of Dracula at the hands of the Crew of Light signifies the triumph of one colonial power over another. For such triumphs to take place, England had to have heroes, and homosexuality was incompatible with colonial notions of manhood and heroism. Hence, it was attributed to the Count. Like the homophobic discourses in all countries, which insist that homosexuality is not native to that land but an undesirable element brought into it by traders, invaders, or immigrants, *Dracula*, too, ascribes homosexuality to a foreigner figure, who spreads it like a disease, and the only willing taker for which is the already unhinged Renfield.

Hemendra Kumar Roy, who had to live and write under a colonial regime, was singularly concerned with articulating an anti-colonial protest in many of his works. In novels like *Suryanagarir Guptadhan*(*The Treasure of the Incas*) and *Neel Sayarer Achinpure*(*The Unknown City of the Blue Depths*), one finds criticism of colonialism in all its forms, with not even the heroes spared when they inflict violence on the native populace of a land they have visited. In *Bishalgarh-er Duhshahsan*, too, the struggle against Rudrapratap subtly takes on anti-colonial dimensions in at least two ways.

Firstly, Rudrapratap is a Rajput, and somebody who is no longer an independent ruler, his kingdom having been taken over by the British (Roy 2005, 6). The British, who had classed the Rajputs as one of the 'martial races' of India (as opposed to, say, the 'non-martial' Bengalis), relied on their services to safeguard the Empire. Maharaja Takht Singh of Marwar, for one, supported the British during the Revolt of 1857, as did the princely states of Rajputana such as Alwar, Bikaner, Bundi, Jaipur and Jodhpur. In describing the role of the Rajput soldiers serving under the British banner, Captain A. H. Bingley wrote:

> Rajputs have served in our ranks from Plassey to the present day (1899). They have taken part in almost every campaign undertaken by the Indian armies. Under Forde they defeated the French at Condore. Under Monro at Buxar they routed the forces of the Nawab of Oudh. Under Lake they took part in the brilliant series of victories which destroyed the power of the Marathas. (Bingley 1986, 20)

The reference to Plassey brings us to another kind of Rajput—the business class of who hailed from the region called Marwar in Rajputana. Exactly a century before the Revolt of 1857, it had been two 'Marwaris', called Jagat Seth and Umi Chand, both bankers, who had betrayed Bengal's last independent ruler, Nawab Siraj-ud-daula, to the British during the Battle of Plassey in 1757, which enabled the British, under Robert Clive, to establish a firm political foothold in India. In his detective novel *Jagatsheth-er Ratnakuthi* (*The Treasure Chamber of Jagat Seth*), Roy has his investigator hero, Jayanta, deliver a stinging tirade against these Indian agents of the British, whose machinations led Bengal, and later, India, to fall under the yoke of foreign rule (Roy 2010, 30). The mention of Rudrapratap's ethnicity, therefore, aligns him with the British. Bishalgarh, Roy writes, is in central India, and the name of this realm is phonetically similar to Ajaigarh and Bijawar, the two *riyasats* in that region that were ruled by Rajput clans, and which were also supportive of the British.

Against this Rajput aristocrat, Roy pits his Bengali heroes, Abinash-babu and Binoy. The British thought little of the Bengalis as a people, as can be seen from Macaulay's words:

> The physical organisation of the Bengalee [sic] is feeble even to effeminacy...His pursuits are sedentary, his limbs delicate, his movements languid. During many ages he has been trampled upon by men of bolder and more hardy breeds. Courage, independence, veracity, are qualities to which his constitution and his situation are equally unfavourable. His mind bears a singular analogy to his body. It is weak even to helplessness for purposes of manly resistance … (Macaulay "Warren Hastings", URL mentioned in 'References')

Roy's works routinely endeavour to challenge this image of the Bengalis via the daring, physically strong, learned heroes, who are no less than the English in any way, and make it a point to speak out against colonial rule. Abinash-babu and Binoy are protagonists in the same mould. Secondly, the British authorities in Kolkata are portrayed as completely ignorant of the fact that the city is under attack from a vampire. As Abinash-babu says, "The police shall not do anything to help us…if we try telling them that a vampire is behind all these deaths, they shall pack us off to a lunatic asylum immediately. We must therefore forget the police and act on our own, with discretion" (Roy 2005, 50. Translation ours).[9] Of course, the

---

[9] It is interesting to see the anti-colonial undertones that bristle in Roy's adaptation of Van Helsing's statement while trying to track down Dracula who has escaped from England in a ship:

British being *unaware* of a vampire's arrival in Kolkata is the more charitable explanation of their inaction over it. The other, more disconcerting possibility is that the British have simply decided to look the other way. Count Dracula is the ruler of his realm in Transylvania, free to do with his subjects as he pleases, not answerable to anyone. Rudrapratap's Bishalgarh, as mentioned before, is now under the aegis of British rule. That Rudrapratap can nonetheless terrorise and feed upon the people there hints at a complicity between him and the British. After all, the understanding between the British and the indigenous ruling class in India was that the latter could do what they wished with their subjects, as long as they paid the revenues to the colonisers and took part in no anti-British activities. Individual and idealistic exceptions apart, the British were uninterested in the welfare of the commoners or in protecting them from the oppression by the landlords and the kings and princes; they were happy to let the local rulers deal with the everyday affairs of their respective domains. In the light of these historical facts, the British administration's complete inaction over Rudrapratap, whether in Bishalgarh or Kolkata, is not surprising. It is symptomatic of the indifference of both the colonial and the local aristocratic rulers towards the well-being of common people. In the context of imperialism, then, Rudrapratap's vampirism becomes a metaphor for something else, namely, the way the ordinary citizens were sucked dry by paying the revenues to the local rulers, who, in turn, paid the British their share of it, and since timely payment to the British was necessary for staying in their good books, the kings and the landlords were ruthless about collecting the taxes from their subjects, who were not spared from paying their dues under any circumstances.

Either because of their cluelessness about the threat that hangs over Kolkata, therefore, or their complicity in it, the British, in *Bishalgarh-er Duhshasan*, do nothing to apprehend Rudrapratap. Hence, it is up to Abinash-babu and Binoy to ensure the safety of their fellow citizens. This, too, is a favoured tactic of Roy's: in his stories, he renders the colonisers

---

"... what is to be done is not for police or of the customs. It must be done by us alone and in our own way." (Stoker, *Dracula*, Norton Critical Edition) 277.

irrelevant by making them ineffectual. In the Jayanta stories, the inspector Sundar-babu, who, as an officer in Calcutta Police, represents the British government, regularly visits Jayanta to seek the latter's assistance for cases that cannot be solved by the authorities, and indeed, it is ultimately Jayanta who finds the culprit who has been eluding the police. This trope may be borrowed from Arthur Conan Doyle's Sherlock Holmes tales, where Lestrade's inefficiency often allows Holmes to prove his calibre as a detective, but when translocated to a colonised land, with indigenous detectives replacing the British one, the trope acquires a different significance.

The queerness in Hemendra Kumar Roy's heroes goes hand-in-hand with their anti-colonialism, indicating that Roy did not find the two to be mutually exclusive. Bimal and Kumar, or Barun and Arun, or for that matter, Abinash-babu and Binoy, are both queer and opposed to colonialism. That Roy should find no contradiction between the two does not come as a surprise to anyone who knows about the Indian freedom movement. Firaq Gorakhpuri, an avowed Gandhian, a participant in the Non-Cooperation Movement of 1922, and a famous Urdu poet, penned a robust rebuttal to an essay by an unnamed critic, published in the journal *Kaleem*, which had criticised the Urdu ghazals for celebrating same-sex love. The response by Gorakhpuri, whose homosexuality was well-known in the circles he moved in, appeared in *Nigaar* in 1936. In it, he cites the many gifted Urdu poets who have celebrated same-sex love, names the western luminaries who are homosexual, and calls the unnamed critic and his ilk "Instruments of instruction for the British government" (Vanita and Kidwai 2000, 265). In other words, he associates the critic's homophobia with British rule—an apt argument, given that Section 377, the law that continues to criminalise all same-sex activity in India, is a remnant of the colonial government. Gopabandhu Das, another Gandhian freedom fighter, wrote a collection of poems called *Poems Written in Prison*, and two of them are characterized by intense romantic longings for his male compatriot (Ibid., 242). Gandhi's own view on homosexuality was that it is an 'unnatural vice' (Ibid., 255), but he did not single it out for condemnation. Rather, his belief in the virtues of celibacy made him denounce *any* sexual desire as a hindrance to the full dedication of one's life to social service and spiritual pursuits. Furthermore, he says that these 'vices' have been a part of human psyche since 'times immemorial' (Ibid.), rather than something brought to Indian shores by the British. Even more interestingly, his disapproval of sexual desire did not prevent him from writing the following letter to Charles Frear Andrews, who, Gandhi says, is in need of 'a curator euphemistically called nurse' (Ibid.), and adds:

> And how I should like to occupy that post! If you cannot have a nurse like me, who would make love to you but at the same time enforce strict obedience to the doctor's orders, you need a wife...But marriage is probably too late. And not being able to nurse you myself I can only fret. (Ibid., 254-55)

Gandhi's correspondence with Hermann Kallenbach, the German-Jewish architect and bodybuilder who was also dedicated to the Indian leader, likewise has sentences like "How completely you have taken possession of my body. This is slavery with a vengeance." They pledged to each other "more love, and yet more love ... (such as) the world has not yet seen" (Lelyveld 2011, 89-90).

Sabbir Hasan Khan, whose poems, written under the name Josh Malihabadi, championed the cause of India's freedom from the British, had admitted in his autobiography *Yaadon Ki Baraat* (*A Procession of Memories*, 1970) that he had fallen in love eighteen times in his life, and on two of those occasions with men. The letters he exchanged with Samad Yar Khan, better known as Saghar Nizami and also a reknowned poet in his own right, bear testimony to the romantic relationship they shared (Katyal 2013, 198).

Subhash Chandra Bose, the celebrated founder-leader of the Indian National Army that fought the British, addressed his fellow freedom fighter Hemanta Kumar Sarkar in a letter dated 22nd May, 1914, with sentences like, "Dear, I just received your letter that you have written with the love-warmed blood of your heart", "Even if you do not ask for it openly, I shall lay at your feet all the love, and a million times more, that my tiny heart can hold", "I beg you, do not forget that I am yours and you are mine, forever", and "You are my Krishna... even if the world castigates you as a sinner, you are my God" (Bose 2007, 29. Translation ours). Krishna, the Hindu deity, is known mostly for his many love affairs with women, but his relationship with the warrior Arjun was no less romantic[10], and there are multiple accounts of Him transforming into the female form of Mohini and making love to other Hindu deities like Shiva. Bose, in calling his beloved male friend "my Krishna", positions both of them within this Hindu queer lore, which, he says, "is mocked by the English-educated youth of today" (Bose 2007, 29. Translation ours). Like Gorakhpuri, Bose associates homophobia with British influence.

As with these freedom fighters, whose fight against the British did not preclude the articulation of the same-sex desires that British law penalised, Roy's heroes are both queer and anti-colonial. This, in fact, is one more way in which Roy removes any trace of pathology from queerness, for if manifested in figures whose opposition to the British is one of the things that make them heroic, it becomes all the more difficult to look upon homosexuality as a perversion of any sort.

One may conclude, then, that Hemendra Kumar Roy is doing something complex with *Bishalgarh-er Duhshasan*. The influence of western literature on him is undeniable. This particular novel is a direct adaptation of a well-known English work, but even in works that are not based on any specific foreign texts, one cannot overlook the affective presence of authors like Edgar Allan Poe, Gaboriau, Maurice Leblanc, and, of course, Conan Doyle, all of whom, in fact, are named in his *Jayanter Kirti* (*The Triumph of Jayanta*). The same work also mentions that Jayanta and his assistant Manik quit college in support of the Non-Cooperation Movement (Roy 2010, 13). The juxtaposition of their love for western detective fiction and their involvement in the Freedom Struggle of India is reflective of Roy's own simultaneous admiration for the works of certain English and European authors and his anti-colonialism. In *Bishalgarh-er Duhshasan*, the same mindset is at work: fascinated by the thrills of

[10] For instance, in the *Padma Purana*, Krishna turns Arjun into a woman named Arjuni and proceeds to make love to Arjuni.

Stoker's novel, Roy adapts it, but not without making alterations that refute the colonialism. His eradication of Stoker's homophobia, and, in particular, of the association of homosexuality with a contagious disease, is part of these alterations too. Rudrapratap may be queer, like Dracula, but so are the heroes, Abinash-babu and Binoy, and since the couple has to fight the vampire sans any help from the British who may well be in league with Rudrapratap, queerness and anti-colonialism are ascribed to the same set of characters. By thus associating a supposed sexual perversion with heroic opposition to foreign rule, Roy attempts to wash off the stigma associated with homosexuality.

SUNIL KUMAR GANGOPADHYAY'S ADAPTATION

Ironically, a second Bengali take on *Dracula*, published eighteen years after *Bishalgarh-er Duhshasan*, opted to follow in the footsteps of Stoker rather than challenge his views the way Roy did. *Bidehi Atma* (*The Disembodied Spirit*, 1967) by Sunil Kumar Gangopadhyay, which appeared in the same year that the British decriminalised homosexuality even as its former colonies (like India) held on to the homophobic laws, replaces Transylvania with the remote regions of Assam, where the fictional realm of Bhishangarh is ruled by Kritanta Barma, the counterpart of Count Dracula.[11] In the fort-like abode of this Assamese vampire, the Bengali Harker, now called Ashoke Lahiri, encounters, not three Brides, but three *male* subordinates of Kritanta Barma, one fair-complexioned and the other two dark. Once the fair one sinks his fangs into Ashoke's throat, the fury of Kritanta Barma takes on a new resonance of jealousy at being upstaged by a subordinate when the Raja drives the threesome away, with the proprietorial, "This man is mine, yes mine!" (Gangopadhyay 1967, 43.

[11] Sunil Kumar Gangopadhyay, *Bidehi Atma, 'The Disembodied Spirit'* (Mandal Book House, Calcutta: 1967). All textual references are to this edition. The name of this vampire and his domain are etymologically significant. 'Kritanta' is another name for the Hindu god of death, *Yama*, who rules the underworld. The surname Barma is the title of a *kshatriya*, a person belonging to the warrior class in the Hindu caste system. 'Bhishan' translates as 'terrible', and 'garh' means fort. See above, the explanation of 'Bishalgarh' 13, fn. 7.

Translation ours) One of the three, far more defiantly than Stoker's or Roy's Brides, shouts back, "Why will only you alone take him? A man has come after so many days – give us our share too." Far more explicitly than Dracula or Rudrapratap, Kritanta Barma says, "Once I get him to do all I want, I will give him to you. Then you can suck blood from his body as you like" (Ibid., 43-44. Translation ours). The second time Ashoke sees them outside his door, Kritanta Barma, like Rudrapratap, and Dracula in the American edition of Stoker's novel, and, again, more explicitly than in either, says, "All the blood tonight is mine. Come tomorrow. Tomorrow's night is allotted to you" (Ibid., 55. Translation ours).

All of this queers Kritanta Barma beyond any scope of doubt, but the trouble lies elsewhere: unlike Roy, where not only the antagonist but also the protagonists are queer, Sunil Kumar Gangopadhyay restricts queerness to the vampiric villains only. The Crew of Light in *Bidehi Atma* is as heterosexual as the one in Stoker's novel, though Gangopadhyay takes a different route to ensure this heterosexuality. Ashoke, the Harker of this book, is portrayed as a married man with a son, and this son, Aloke, is the Mina Harker figure here. This has the result of assuring readers that Ashoke is heterosexual (unlike the unmarried Binoy in Roy, with his attachment to an older man, Abinash-babu). Besides, by rendering this heterosexual character's son vulnerable to the queer Kritanta Barma, homosexuality is turned into a threat that must be eliminated for the sake of heterosexual marriage and parenthood to survive. Similarly, Lucy is turned into Shibu, the younger brother of Tarun, the Arthur Holmwood counterpart. Tarun and Shibu's mother is also present among the characters in the novel, thus ensuring that this too is a 'normal', heterosexual household which, like Ashoke's, is under threat from the queer vampire. Thus, when Ashoke, Tarun, Arup Kar (John Seward), Sanatan Mitra (Quincey Morris) and Shankar Chakrabarti (Van Helsing) come together to rescue Aloke from the vampires, the three latter men become, presumably, surrogate uncles to the young boy, who must be stopped from being seduced into queerness/vampirism.

Even more unfortunately, Gangopadhyay seems to have entirely internalised Stoker's nineteenth-century view of homosexuality as pathology. The victims of Kritanta Barma, like those of Dracula, become vampires themselves; worse still, they seem to prey only on members of their own sex, thus strengthening the image of the homosexual as a violent figure who attempts to swell his cabal by seduction, coercion and transformation. Shibu, after being vampirised, is reported to be feeding on both boys and girls (Ibid., 99) but we see him attack only boys (Ibid., 102-106). Furthermore, Shankar Chakrabarti and Arup Kar are, like Van Helsing and Seward, doctors, and their expertise is sought in the fight against the queer vampires, which only underscores the influence of the medical model of homosexuality that influenced Stoker, and, it is obvious, Gangopadhyay too. Renfield also shows up in *Bidehi Atma* under the name Binayak, who similarly utters rhapsodies about Kritanta Barma. Therefore, in this adaptation, the warring sides are those of 'healthy', heterosexual men, and 'diseased' queer ones, and the outcome is a foregone conclusion. Strangely, Gangopadhyay includes a belated appearance by the three Brides of the vampire towards the end of the book, which means it is unlikely that he turned Mina and Lucy into boys merely to keep his work free of heterosexual seduction scenes. The Brides in this adaptation may address Aloke as "brother" (Ibid., 160), but like the use of the term "sister" by Dracula's Brides to address Mina, the feelings expressed are hardly fraternal/sororial.

Gangopadhyay is so singularly focussed on Kritanta Barma's queerness that he is unable to add any more dimensions to the character. Since the book is set in the 1960s, and the action spread across Assam and Bengal, the tensions and clashes between the Assamese and Bengali-speaking communities that was taking place at the time could have possibly added a fascinating subtext to the tale of an Assamese vampire and the Bengali Crew of Light fighting to bring him down. But for Gangopadhyay, Assam seems to be no more than a mysterious, quasi-exotic setting (much as Transylvania was to Stoker and his fellow countrymen in the nineteenth century), and consequently, Kritanta Barma's ethnicity turns out to have no separate significance. *Bidehi Atma* has little interest in using the vampire figure's background to offer some insight into the socio-political circumstances of the era it was written in, in contrast with the way Roy uses Rudrapratap's Rajput ancestry to tacitly address the camaraderie of interest between the British and the Indian ruling class, or even the way Stoker aligns the Count with Russia to remind his readers of the threat that country posed to Britain's colonial interests. The contrast with Roy's work is notable in other ways as well. Rudrapratap's villainy stems from the fact that he kills, and that he is in league with the colonisers, neither of which has much to do with his sexual proclivities. But as Kritanta Barma's bite spreads his 'affliction' instead of claiming the victims' lives, and since little is made of his being Assamese and no commentary, subtle or prominent, offered about the perils of parochialism as manifested in the then-raging Bengali-Assamese conflict, it is his queerness that attracts the maximum attention, and hence becomes the defining tenet of his villainy.

This proves, more than anything else, that belonging to a newer generation or writing in the later half of the twentieth century does not guarantee progressive thinking. *Bidehi Atma* is dedicated to three men, one of whom is Amiya Kumar Chakrabarti, to whom Hemendra Kumar Roy dictated – on account of pen cramp – *Bishalgarh-er Duhshasan*, and who subsequently published it from his publishing house Abhyuday Prakash Mandir (Roy 1992, foreword). It is possible, then, to assume that Gangopadhyay had read Roy's adaptation, and found the latter's embrace of homosexuality a bit too much to bear. Little else explains his fastidious adherence to the homophobic tenets of Stoker's original.

CONCLUSION

A possible objection to the reading of *Bishalgarh-er Duhshasan* and *Bidehi Atma* as as more queer-friendly and more homophobic versions respectively of *Dracula* could be that the homoeroticism in Roy or the homophobia in Gangopadhyay is merely an inadvertent outcome of de-sexing the source-text for younger readers by removing Lucy and Mina. Human females in *Bidehi Atma* consist of the nurse(s) in Arup Roy's hospital, Shibu's mother, and the nameless girl being stalked by Kritanta

Barma at Sodepur (Gangopadhyay 1967, 94). On the supernatural side, there is the sudden appearance of three Brides of the vampire towards the end (noted above). None of this in any way lessens the homophobic implications of the changes Gangopadhyay makes to his source. Unfortunately, as we have been unable to locate any other work by Gangopadhyay, we are unable to place our conclusions in the larger context of his output.

But much of the voluminous work of Roy can be accessed, helping one to assess the overall bent of his works, including those for younger readers. He was rarely a stickler for the so-called 'rules' regarding books aimed at this demographic. Many Bengali authors believed that children's books should have minimal violence. Roy's works, such as *Bibhishaner Jagaran* (*A Terror Awakens*), *Mrityu-Mallar* (*The Tune of Death*), and *Amabasyar Raat* (*New-Moon Nights*) are all awash with gore. Heterosexual romantic entanglements, too, find their way into *Chhatrapati-r Chhora* (*The Dagger of Shivaji*), and *Runu-Tunu-r Adventure* (*The Adventures of Runu and Tunu*), in yet another 'violation' of the said rules. In the four novels he wrote for the *Bichitra* Series, all adaptations of foreign thrillers/detective novels, he retains the sexual dynamics of his sources. Be it Dr Watson and Mary Morston's romance in *The Sign of Four*, or the triangle of Henry Baskerville and the Stapleton couple in *The Hound of the Baskervilles*, Roy does not shy away from including any of it in *Chaturbhujer Swakshar* and *Nishachari Bibhishika* respectively. In *Guptadhaner Duswapna* (*Nightmare of Treasure*) there is even a full-blown kissing scene.

The homoeroticism in Roy, therefore, is likely more deliberate than accidental, much like the violence and the heterosexual liaisons. Considered in conjunction with the more explicit references to homosexuality in his adult novels (See above, 12), the most legitimate conclusion to arrive at, on the basis of the contents of *Bishalgarh-er Duhshasan*, is that subverting the homophobia of Stoker was part of Roy's stated aim of updating an 'outdated novel'.

References

(Only those works from which quotations have been given, or to which there are close references, have been listed)

Primary Texts

Stoker, Bram. *Dracula* (1897) 1997. Edited by Nina Auerbach and David J. Skal. New York: W.W. Norton and Company.

Roy, Hemendra Kumar. 1949, rpt. 1964. *Bishalgarh-er Duhshasan.* Kolkata: Abhyuday Prakashana Mandir.

Roy, Hemendra Kumar. 2005. *Bishalgarh-er Duhshasan.* In *Hemendra Kumar Roy Rachanabali, vol. 18*. Kolkata: Asia Publishing Company.

Roy, Hemendra Kumar. 2005. *Kuber Purir Rahasya*. In *Hemendra Kumar Roy Rachanabali, vol. 18*. Kolkata: Asia Publishing Company.

Roy, Hemendra Kumar. 2010. *Jagatsheth-er Ratnakuthi.* In *Hemendra Kumar Roy Rachanabali, vol. 25*. Kolkata: Asia Publishing Company, 2010.

Roy, Hemendra Kumar. 1987. *Jayanter Kirti*. In *Hemendra Kumar Roy Rachanabali, vol. 10*. Kolkata: Asia Publishing Company.

Gangopadhyay, Sunil Kumar. 1967. *Bidehi Atma.* Kolkata: Mandal Book House.

Bose, Subhash Chandra. 2007. *Netaji Subhashchandra Basu-r Aprakashita Patrabali*, edited by Abul Ahsan Chowdhury. Dhaka: Shobha Prakash.

Secondary Texts

Bingley, A. H. 1986. *Handbook on Rajputs*. New Delhi: Asian Educational Services.

Brady, Sean. 2014. "Homosexuality: European and Colonial Encounters", in *A Cultural History of Sexuality in the Age of Empire*, edited by Chiara Beccalossi and Ivan Crozier. London: Bloomsbury Academic.

Craft, Christopher. 1997. ""Kiss Me with Those Red Lips": Gender and Inversion in Bram Stoker's *Dracula*", in Stoker, *Dracula* Norton Critical Edition, edited by Nina Auerbach and David J. Skal 444-59. New York: W.W. Norton and Company.

Herdt, Gilbert. 1998. *Same Sex, Different Cultures: Gays and Lesbians across Cultures* Colorado: Westview Press.

Katyal, Akhil. 2013. "Gay Writing and the Idea of Doubleness", in *Masculinity and its Challenges in India: Essays on Changing Perceptions*, edited by Rohit. K. Dasgupta and K. Moti Gokulsing. 187-200. Jefferson: McFarland and Company, Inc., Publishers.

Lelyveld, Joseph. 2011. *Great Soul: Mahatma Gandhi and his Struggle with India*. New York: Vintage.

Macaulay, Thomas Babington. "Warren Hastings." Accessed 23 May 2016 http://www.columbia.edu/itc/mealac/pritchett/00generallinks/macaulay/hastings/txt_complete.html.

Makowski, John F. 2014. "Greek Love in the Greek Novel", in *A Companion to the Ancient Novel*, edited by Edmund P. Cueva and Shannon N. Byrne. New Jersey: Wiley Blackwell.

Mottier, Veronique. 2008. *Sexuality: A Very Short Introduction.* London: Oxford University Press.

Nandy, Mridul. 'Language Movement in Barak Valley, 19 May 1961: An Era of Brave Bengali Revolution'. Accessed 22 May, 2016.http://mridul-nandy.blogspot.in/2012/04/language-movement-in-barak-valley-19.html.

Schaffer, Talia. 1997. '"A Wilde Desire Took Me": The Homoerotic History of *Dracula*', in Stoker, *Dracula,* Norton Critical Edition, edited by Nina Auerbach and David J. Skal. 470-82. New York: W.W. Norton and Company.

Skal, David J. 2014. *Hollywood Gothic: The Tangled Web of Dracula from Novel to Stage to Screen.* New York: W.W. Norton and Company.

Towlson, Jon. 2016. *The Turn to Gruesomeness in American Horror Films, 1931-1936* Jefferson: McFarland and Company, Inc., Publishers.

Vanita, Ruth and Saleem Kidwai, ed. 2000. *Same-Sex Love in India: Readings in Indian Literature.* New York: Palgrave Macmillan.

In: Imperial Maladies
Editors: D. Bandyopadhyay et al.
ISBN: 978-1-53611-863-6

Chapter 11

THE CENTRE AND ITS MIRROR: CASE STUDIES OF FOURTH WORLD POISONS AS A MOTIF IN COLONIAL BENGAL'S DETECTIVE FICTION

Piali Mondal*
Department of English, Jadavpur University, Kolkata, West Bengal, India

To say that the Fourth World poison was a favoured motif in the empire's narratives of mystery and detection would be an understatement, as the trope ran its whole gamut from the blow-pipes and poisoned darts in the Sherlock Holmes murder mysteries to the Christie intrigues about curare. The reasons for its allure are not entirely unrelated to the Empire and anxieties, and a bulk of such reasons, though not all, are connected to the empire's fascination with the Fourth World itself.

*Corresponding Author's Email: iluvmizukamishin@gmail.com.

As Greenblatt mentions in his seminal essay "Invisible Bullets," the first step of culturally assimilating and overpowering a conquered people is stratification of knowledge. However, the appropriation is made harder when there is no physical evidence of that which is to be appropriated, that is, cultural information. In absence of books, scrolls, or other sources of information which can be pilfered, the only possible way of documenting oral culture is, of course, via communication with the indigene. A further need for such information may be a fear of cultural assimilation that the empire itself feels as its boundary increases, and, in such situations, a bonafide citizen of the empire who considers herself to be at the centre of it, should, naturally feel the need to distinguish her from the "other." The poisoned darts work so well as a motif, because, in the hand of a discerning writer, they hold the capacity to both titillate and abate such anxieties. They stand as a symbol of infiltrations of two kinds; firstly, that of an object of heretofore unknown origins infiltrating and disrupting a "civilised" society, and, secondly, that of said society being corrupted from within, as it is often found in such fictions that the applier of the poison is not someone from the place where it originates, but, rather, from the country of the reader, or from a country with a similar civilisation; a native accomplice, if any, is shown as a lackey working in compliance with the rules set up by a civilised perpetrator.

This was a rough estimation of the methods the motif uses to titillate the reader representing the empire, and the execution and closing of the story is what abates or tries to abate such anxieties when they arise. The poison motif is something the skilled writer could and did use to both ends. A poisoned dart, though a symbol of the savage people that exist within the empire, is a visible and quantifiable entity, and is always accompanied by an anecdotal passage within the work itself, ideally uttered by the detective himself/ herself. This passage both stratifies and alienates the information about the poison, so that the poison becomes both "known" and the "other," a weapon potentially outlandish and harmful, but, nevertheless, identifiable and controllable. Furthermore, the culpability of the criminal working from within the empire, while increasing the anxiety of corruption, represents a rational, and, like the poison, an identifiable entity.

A disruption caused by a rational mind, as the narratives of mystery and detection dictate, may well be stopped by another rational mind, in this case that of the well-informed sleuth. Thus, the Fourth World poison in colonial detective fiction is presented as a potentially harmful enigma, but an enigma that can, nevertheless, be contained and solved.

However, even the method by which the motif is incorporated into the narrative will differ from the centre to the further colonies, though there are bound to be certain similarities. An author from the colonies, who puts his work up for popular publication, can be seen as mirroring his British counterparts in more ways than one. For one, the early sleuths of colonial Bengal were penned by men of well to moderate means who had received a standard amount of westernised education, had leisure to write about dare-devil chases from the comforts of home, and, last but not the least, were well attuned to the centre's desire for law and order in the colonies. This was augmented by the fact that this was a genre heretofore unexplored in the literature of colonial Bengal, so the writers, naturally, drew some inspiration from the European, and, most commonly, the British writers.

What, then, is the basis for differences we see in the treatment of the poison motif, when the works of a British writer and a Bengali writer from the empire are compared? Here is where another aspect of both the aforementioned "mirror" and the "mirror" of the title comes in. The image produced by a mirror, while seemingly identical, is always reversed. Similarly, the writer and the reader of colonial Bengal are posited in the power-structure of the empire in a way that mirrors the position of the British writer and the British reader, the aforementioned similarities making them more aware of the mirrored reversal. They, like the reader at the centre of the empire, are also experiencing cultural schizophrenia, but the ideas of the self and the other are blurred to such an extent that the intent to be faithful to either becomes ambivalent. This ambivalence extends to the writer's concept about the Fourth World too; while the British writer would, and could, only sympathise, the writer from the colony could also empathise with a Fourth World about the disempowerment they both experience, though the degrees and effects of disempowerment are different; however, unlike a member of the Fourth

World, they have a voice, a voice which, nevertheless, is both made possible and controlled by the empire, and the sleuth's responsibility, ultimately, must lie with the civilisation that sustains his existence. The goal of the paper is to examine such ambivalences through a few case studies of the detective fiction of colonial Bengal and its relation, if any, to its British counterpart, and for this purpose a few works by exactly one author from each category has been chosen, as it will allow for a less diverse but hopefully more focussed process of observation. The authors whose works we shall discuss in the paper are Arthur Conan Doyle and Hemendra Kumar Roy.

The reasons for selecting this pair is that, aside from being the trendsetters in detective fiction of their respective cultures, they seem to have a keen ear for public demand, as well as a visible similarity of ethical temperament. Such similarities make it easier for us to notice differences, if any. Moreover, as it has been said about Hemendra Kumar Roy that, plot-wise, he was heavily dependent on western fiction, this seems to be an occasion that may be able to shed light on the veracity of that claim. The works to be discussed are Doyle's *The Sign of Four* and "The Adventure of the Sussex Vampire," and Roy's *Choturbhujer Swakhkhar* (1956), "Agadh Joler Rui-Katla" or 'Deep-Water Fish'(1940) *and Shani-Mangaler Rahasya* or *The Saturn-Mars Mystery.* All of them discuss a specific method of poisoning, that is, dart-poisoning.

A prudent way to start would be with *Choturbhujer Swakhkhar* and *The Sign of Four*, as the former is a more or less faithful adaptation of the latter. However, as has been mentioned before, the Bengali writer of the colonies and the British writer writing from the core of the empire are bound to have different approaches to this topic, and such differences must be brought to the fore. One of the principal differences is, of course, the time in which they were written. For this, and for the cultural differences, the poisoner from the Fourth World, that is, Tonga, the Andamanese aborigine, becomes slightly different creatures in the two narratives. Doyle, of course, writes in the heyday of the empire, and it is hardly surprising that he would give such a description of Tonga: "They are a fierce, morose, and intractable people, though capable of forming most devoted friendships when their confidence has once been gained". (Doyle 1890, 30) Furthermore, after adding how "Naturally hideous" (Doyle 1890, 30) they are, Holmes goes on to put deliberate emphasis on their intractability, "So intractable and fierce they are that all the efforts of the British officials to win them over have failed". (Doyle 1890, 30) After adding to this a brief and gruesome description of Tonga's tribe's cannibalism, Holmes concludes by saying, "Watson! If this fellow had been left to his own unaided devices this affair might have taken an even more ghastly turn". (Doyle 1890, 30) This seems to ratify our earlier point that a savage man held in check by a white man, who is a more "rational" accomplice, was a device used by the narrative to ensure that the disruption caused by their activities would be contained, and the whiteness, or, at the very least, the presence of a civilised villain, was considered a desirable quality, as a rational person, unlike a man such as the one trained to commit all the horrors described in the gazetteer Holmes reads, can, and will, ultimately be dealt with another rational person, in this case, the sleuth. However, Hemendra Kumar Roy's adaptation dates back to 1956, the only work in our selection that was written in independent India, and, as has been proven by Roy's fierce defence of the native Americans and the thorough condemnation of the white colonisers in *Rakta Patharer Santaru*, or *Swimmer in the Ocean of Blood,* Roy has an altogether different take on colonisation, and it shows in the manner in which he describes Tonga and the poisoning. Tonga's "natural hideousness" is passed over, and, as any fond reader of Roy would certify, Roy does not shy away from forming a Platonic association between an ugly face and an ugly and uncouth disposition (point in case being the character of Bhairabi in *Runu-Tunur Adventure*). (Roy 2006, 50) There is no comment, either, on the habitual cannibalism of his tribe. His fierceness and intractability is not accompanied with a wistful comment which regrets that he and his tribe could not be won over, nor does the sleuth Bharat feel the need to consult a gazetteer, a symbol of written and reliable information in the original, to describe Tonga and his motives. Furthermore, a small incident is added in which Bharat discovers the rest of Tonga's darts within a basket of mixed-colour weaves, an article immediately identified as the workmanship of basket-weavers in central India. This may be a mere coincidence, but it also makes for a reduction of the alien aspect of Tonga, and, moreover connects his narrative to the Indian mainland, and therefore he cannot be put in the same category with the frightful and almost spectral Tonga described by Doyle.

"The Adventure of the Sussex Vampire" and *Shani Mangaler Rahasya or The Saturn-Mars Mystery,* are similar in the sense that they can be seen as exercises to understand the peril of sensationalising the "other." In the first case, the county of Sussex seems to have imported an otherworldly mystery from Peruvia: a mother and wife, who, while seemingly devoted to her husband and child, is willing to feed on her son to satisfy her vampiric urges. Her "alien religion" (Doyle 1924, 2) is ominous, and an addition to the suspect's criminal history, that of having violently beaten her step-son, is made by her own husband Mr. Ferguson.The wound via which the South American poison, possibly curare, enters the body, escapes the notice of both the nurse and the husband, who find it a more likely possibility that someone of Peruvian origin may harbour a nefarious tendency or a sickness. Similarly, in *Shani Mangaler Rahasya,* the criminal uses the superstitions prevalent in colonial Bengal to disguise his identity, to the effect that the police officer Sundar babu, who is supposed to be the civilised world's representative of law and order, finds a supernatural force demanding human sacrifice on auspicious days more likely than a human murderer. The revelation of the criminals, however, proves the futility of such superstitions; in 'The Sussex Vampire,' the disfigured boy who is much loved by his father and certainly held to be more reliable and truthful than the vampire, is revealed to be the criminal who applied the poison, and his Oedipal attachment to his dead mother and (possibly) to also his father, is outlined by Holmes to be the root cause for his jealous deeds,(Ibid., 8) and, interestingly, Holmes confirms his suspicion about the boy's culpability by way of a mirrored surface: "I watched him as you fondled the child just now. His face was clearly reflected in the glass of the window where the shutter formed a background. I saw such jealousy, such cruel hatred, as I have seldom seen in a human face." (Doyle 1924, 7) The physical act of poisoning, here, may itself be a metaphor for the poisoning or moral corruption that occurs from within the civilised British society, a poisoning which could be easily overlooked in favour of finding an "other" to indict. Similarly, in *Shani Mangaler Rahasya or The Saturn-Mars Mystery*, the perpetrator is revealed to be Mahendra babu, whose affable smile and genial behaviour had taken in everybody but the sleuth himself, to the effect that the Bornean connection got nearly overlooked. The poison, here, is *ipo*, a deadly plant extract used by the Malay aborigines, which Jayanta identifies by no quality of its own, but by the medium through which it is applied, which is a sago wood dart. The wielder of the poison, as it is revealed later, is Mahendra babu's faithful Bornean driver Ali, but his act is controlled by the seemingly innocuous Mahendra babu, who does not only get Ali to kill his cousin to obtain his property, but also, has two more people murdered for no other reason than to sustain the myth of the Saturday-Tuesday human sacrifices to the goddess Kali, near whose temple all the deaths occur. Mahendra babu's plan, then, is not only dependent on his trusty servant and his skills with the *sumpitan*, but also on the willingness of the locals to keep believing in the superstition. The outcome and intention, though achieving a similar effect of disguise, differ from 'The Sussex Vampire', in that the locals, unlike Ferguson who was only afraid of and repelled by his wife's supposed preternatural affliction, revere the source causing the apparent supernatural deaths. Thus, for them, looking for a possible scientific explanation is not something that they *do not* explore, but also something that they *cannot* explore, the very idea of finding rational explanations for preternatural (or, in this case, divine) activities being alien to their cultural ethos. This is an aspect in which Roy's "other" will always differ from the "other" of Doyle – in a culture so heavily reliant on myth and superstition, the "other" would, very consciously, be a part of the "self."

The device *sumpitan* and the poison *ipo* appear at least once more, in a Bimal-Kumar venture called "Agadh Joler Rui-Katla," 'Deep-Water Fish'. Unlike Jayanta, Bimal and Kumar are not strictly detectives, but, rather, investigators in the broadest sense of that word. They do sometimes act as sleuths, but depending on the demands exacted by their ventures they are most often treasure-hunters (in their first adventure, *Jaker Dhan, 'Haunted*

Treasure,' published in 1930, and in four more of their subsequent exploits), paranormal investigators (*Amabasyar Raat* or *Night of the New Moon,* published in 1939), and unwilling explorers of the cosmos (*Meghduter Martye Agomon,* or *'Advent of the Cloud Messenger'*). Therefore, it is significant that Roy would feature them and the poison in specifically a detective story, and more surprisingly, Sundar babu, who appears in both *Shani Mangaler Rahasya* and "Agadh Joler Rui-Katla," shows no cognition of the poison and its method prior to the explanation in the short story, the events of which take place after those of the novel. Moreover, the motives are similar; the culprits involved were closest successors to properties with no direct heir, and they are not primary suspects on account of the friendship or devotion they had shown to the victims up to the time of their deaths. Considering the stark similarities in motives and modus operandi (and the attempt to treat the adventures as unique and unrelated), this may be Roy's way of making a statement not unconnected to the general effect of the events in "The Adventure of the Sussex Vampire," that is, the corruption and the moral deviance we associate with an alien culture may also be present at the heart of the culture we call our own.

Also, as a final thought, we may recall the identical way in which Jayanta in *Shani Mangaler Rahasya* and Bimal in "Agadh Joler Rui-Katla" emphasise that their knowledge about *ipo* and *sumpitan* comes from a trip to Borneo. Upon catching Ali, the Bornean murderer, Jayanta says, "Ali, don't mess with us. We, too, have been to Borneo." (Roy 2014, 192) Similarly, Bimal in "Agadh Joler Rui-katla" affirmatively answers Sundar babu's query about any past trip to Borneo.(Roy 2014, 127) This insistence on being a widely-travelled person is very alien to the Holmes stories, as the British sleuth rarely has to leave Britain for his cases, and, as seen in *The Sign of Four,* relies on textual sources for information on the remote parts. This sets our Bengali sleuths them apart from Doyle's detective. Their first-hand knowledge of the *ipo* and the *sumpitan*, furthermore, does not let them remain at a distance from the Fourth World. The "othering" is still present, as there is bound to be some similarities in a genre that is not perfectly indigenous, but it also allows and encourages social contact with the "other," and does not value the contact in the terms of quantifiable, and, thus, controllable information it may provide, and therein lies the difference between the centre and its mirror.

REFERENCES

Doyle, Arthur Conan. 1924. "The Adventure of the Sussex Vampire." Accessed 10th October, 2016. https://sherlock-holm.es/stories/pdf/a4/1-sided/suss.pdf.

Doyle, Arthur Conan. 1890. *The Sign of the Four*. Accessed 9th October, 2016. https://sherlock-holm.es/stories/pdf/a4/1-sided/sign.pdf.

Greenblatt, Stephen. 1988. "Invisible Bullets." *'Shakespearean Negotiations: Circulation of Social Energy in Renaissance England'*. California: University of California Press.

Roy, Hemendra Kumar.1976, rpt. 2014. *Amabasyar Rat*. *'Hemendra Kumar Roy Rochonaboli'*. Vol. 2, Kolkata: Asia Publishing Company.

Roy, Hemendra Kumar. 1996, rpt. 2014. "Agadh Joler Rui-Katla." Chhayakayar Mayapure. *Hemendra Kumar Roy Rochonaboli.* Vol.14, Kolkata: Asia Publishing Company.

Roy, Hemendra Kumar. 2006. *Choturbhujer Swakhkhar. Hemendra Kumar Roy Rochonaboli.* Vol. 21, Kolkata: Asia Publishing Company,

*Roy, Hemendra Kumar.*1974, rpt. 2012. *Jakher Dhan. Hemendra Kumar Roy Rochonaboli.* Vol. 1, Kolkata: Asia Publishing Company,

Roy, Hemendra Kumar. 1974, rpt. 2012. *Meghduter Martye Agomon. Hemendra Kumar Roy Rochonaboli.* Vol.1, Kolkata:Asia Publishing Company.

Roy, Hemendra Kumar, 2014. *Rokto patharer Santaru. Hemendra Kumar Roy Rochonaboli.* Vol.28, Kolkata: Asia Publishing Company.

Roy, Hemendra Kumar. 2006. *Runu-Tunur Adventure. Hemendra Kumar Roy Rochonaboli.* Vol.21, Kolkata: Asia Publishing Company.

Roy, Hemendra Kumar. 1976, rpt. 2014. *Shani Mangaler Rohosyo. Hemendra Kumar Roy Rochonaboli.* Vol.2, Kolkata: Asia Publishing Company.

PART 5.
MEDICINE, GENDER AND COLONIAL MODERNITY

In: Imperial Maladies
Editors: D. Bandyopadhyay et al.
ISBN: 978-1-53611-863-6

Chapter 12

WOMEN OF STEEL AMIDST TROPICAL MALADIES

*Suchismita Neogi**
Department of English, Budge Budge College, Kolkata,
West Bengal, India

INTRODUCTION

The late 19th and early 20th century English literary sphere saw the flourishing of both fictional and non-fictional texts written about women by women themselves. Memoirs and travelogues emerged along with other colonial discourses that sketched the social life of the British in India. Flora Annie Steel, born in 1847 England, as E.F. Oaten remarks is "perhaps the greatest novelist in the strictest sense" (Powell 1981, 78) of Anglo-Indian fiction.She came to India at the age of twenty with her husband who was an ICS official then and had his postings in extremely remote areas.The conditions, in which she had to live in India at first, were immensely disturbing. "The heat was terrific. Rain had fallen short, a

*Corresponding author's email: suchismita.bunan@gmail.com.

famine was threatening, especially in the Cis-Sutlej districts of the Panjab, through which we were literally whirled in the box upon wheels, drawn by miserable starveling ponies, which at that time was the only method of travel beyond Delhi" (Steel 1929, 30).

Sometimes Steel was the only European woman in her region and thus, she made her decision of learning the local languages and "acquiring knowledge of India and its people" with the intention of "learning more or less how to manage them" (Steel 1929, 52). The non-fictional works of Steel, especially her autobiography, *The Garden of Fidelity* (1929) expose her profound approval for the imperialist endeavours in India.She advocated an authoritarian attitude towards the natives believing in "the absolute necessity for high-handed dignity in dealing with those who for thousand years have been accustomed to it" (Steel 1929, 133). Steel felt that the insurgence was brought to an end by the Indians due to a psychological factor which made them willingly dominated by the British masters. Like most Europeans, she also considered Indians to be effeminate and sensual. For her, the natives were like children who needed and wanted to be mastered. Surprisingly, she was also critical about the role of the British rulers in the revolt and had remarked, "If ever a race brought revolt on itself, we did so, in India" (Steel 1909, 195). She even described the Empire's policy of forceful acquirement of Awadh as "mean in the extreme" sense (Steel 1929, 350). Again, contradicting herself, she blamed Bentick for his "tinkering with the Indian law" (Steel 1929, 346) with his amendatory policies regarding Sati, female education and the activities of proselytisation as well. At the same time, she also belittles the participation of the natives in the mutiny by defining their motive as mere "lust of power." Steel even points out that only a small part of the populace was involved in the revolt while the major portion, which consisted mostly of the peasantry, "dreamt on peacefully"(Steel 1929, 353).

During these times, considerable emphasis was given on the representation of the native woman as an attempt of providing them an identity of the "other." Reformist issues worked in favour of the improvement of women's status, and during such endeavours, the idea of the 'exotic woman' was seen to be an extra addition to the white man's burden of imperialist "anxieties." The rulers portrayed themselves as humane reformists intending to free the native women from the shackles of brothels and other patriarchal modes of exploitation. So it can be said that the issue of "social reforms" was indeed very complicated.Though the colonialists actually helped to bring an end to several social evils, their reformative policies became a licence for the continuation of the British Raj in the country. Mrs. E.J. Chapman minutely observes the role of the British masters in fighting against sati and also in passing an Anti-Sati Legislation in 1829. Steel's narratives also often speak of the horrors of female infanticide.She even talks about the practice in detail by describing the actions of rural Panjab women who would leave their new born girl child outside their village to be carried off by jackals. But it is interesting to note that none of the writings of the 'memsahibs' elaborate upon or even mention the role of Indian reformers who actively participated in the campaigns against the dominating social curses.

Steel's long stay of almost twenty two years in India helped her to reveal the heart and soul of the natives through her works. She attempted to bring forth the complicated lives of the Anglo-Indian women who had to survive in colonial India. The status of a conventional Memsahib was gradually subdued once Steel acquired interest in the day-to-day lives of the natives, especially the women. She was given the title of "Female Kipling" for her contributions to colonial discourses but her attitude towards the natives did not assert Kipling's agenda in which he tried to hint that females were a misfit in the colony. However, the new avatar of the "unconventional Memsahib" was not enough to free Steel from the stigma of being an Imperialist and neither did she make amends to cleanse her portraiture. It has often been stated that though she had become thoroughly involved with the lives of the natives, their social issues and also voiced protests against the oppression of their women, she never deferred from her image of the British coloniser. Though Steel belonged to the group of "memsahib writers," her works were very different from her contemporaries. *The Spectator* had commented her to be a "sympathetic and acute interpreter of the native life in India" (*The Spectator* 20 June 1903, 984). The birth of her daughter gave Steel the chance to interact with the natives at a closer proximity. She mentions in her autobiography several accounts of her daughter's ayah named Fazli. She wholeheartedly praises Fazli for being better than English nurses in terms of order, discipline and most importantly cleanliness. Though Steel held a firm opinion about the English nurse being a lot better than the native ones but in this case, Fazli wins her over.

Her stay at Kasur helped her most to understand Indian ways and also to grasp the Indian mentality to a certain extent. As Steel mentions in her autobiography, *The Garden of Fidelity*, "At Kasur there was literally no one but the natives" (Steel 1929, 104) and thus she undertook the duties of a reformer and started to take care of sick Indian women and children and also taught English to some interested scholars. Despite her reformative propagandas, she faced extreme difficulties in "educating India on Western lines while the environment remained Eastern" (Steel 1929, 62-63). In the year 1889, Flora Annie Steel left India and returned back to Britain where a friend suggested her to write some more about her experiences in colonial estate. She obeyed and her novel, *Miss Stuart's Legacy* along with many other stories was successfully published by the Macmillan's. Steel kept coming back to India for her researches before the completion of each of her other books such as *On the Face of the Waters* and *Voices in the Night*. Her novels contain a varied range of female characters beyond the conventional memsahib. Her novel, *The Hosts of the Lords*, for example revolve around the interconnected stories of Erda, the Scotswoman and Laila, the Eurasian woman and their attempts to escape marriage. Steel's male characters too, show notable variations as in the case of Dick Smith in *Miss Stuart's Legacy*. The character, as often depicted by postcolonial critics, is a hybridised form of both the Indian and the British and in the process of oscillating between these two completely opposite identities, disturb the hierarchies of the colonial society. The Eurasians were unanimously smirked at by both the coloniser and the colonised and even the authors belonging to the class of white people hinted at the social and racial inferiority of such mixed blood. Beneath all the contempt and ridicule that was meted out to the Eurasians, was perhaps, the latent doubt amongst the colonisers that feared people of mixed races where a potential threat to the distinctions between the ruler and the ruled.

Steel planned to write a book about the Mutiny in India and thus in the year 1894, she returned to the subcontinent with all available details about the revolt. She mentions in her autobiography that during her stay, she did a lot of doctoring, sometimes, having over fifty patients a day and at the same time talked to the natives about their views and personal reflections on the mutiny. She narrates her action to be similar as "digging for gold, uncertain each instant if some priceless treasure would not turn up. And there was a breathless haste, an inevitable hurry about it, almost as if the spirit of the times had been caught and prisoned" (Steel 1929, 214). *On the Face of the Waters* ultimately emerged as a multi-dimensional novel with notable contributions in various aspects. The question, whether the book can be used as an authentic, unbiased source of historical evidence of the mutiny is debatable but Steel's concept of the "new woman" which we find in the same narrative is undoubtedly a product of fertile intelligentsia.

The novel challenges the predominant Victorian ideals in respect to race and gender by highlighting the complicated habitat in which the presumed racially superior "white women" were subjected to gendered subordination. Kate Erlton, Steel's protagonist and Alice Gissing, Major Erlton's mistress are the representatives of the diverse physical and intellectual positioning of the Anglo-Indian women. Steel uses Kate as the trunk for her gynocentric narrative, a genre that was rare in colonial fiction. The novel traces the journey of Kate from the British "home culture" into that of the colonised state. Her attitude towards English practices and wilful adoption of the Indian ones facilitate her survival during the mutiny but seclude her from her co-Britons. Her venture outside the home culture allows her to rise beyond the subjugating English expectations. This home culture can be said to be intentionally created by the Britons to assert a cultural and moral superiority in the psychology of both the coloniser and the colonised. The women were just a medium of envisaging "authentic" English nationalism; their bodies and their culture, a reminder of the Empire's importance for the rulers residing in the colonised states.

The English women in these colonies portray a very critical situation in terms of identity – where they were both the dominating and the dominated cult. Kate, as a coloniser exercises control over the natives while at the same time, suffers indelibly under a philandering husband and also an oppressive Victorian culture. According to Steel, Indian womanhood was the epitome of "the greatest amount self-abnegation" (Steel 1905, 159) and thus validated the notion of submissive and self-sacrificing women. Kate, at first, can be seen as a reflection of such idealistic belief that considered marriage to be a solemn religious duty. However, Alice Gissing's attitudes towards such social morals stand in opposition. She lives a free life and unlike Kate, does not let the strict English rules captivate her. Unfortunately, it is Alice who becomes one of the first victims of the Mutiny that breaks out on 11th May in Delhi. May be, Steel found this to be a way of 'redeeming' a sexually active Victorian Woman as she considered that the origin of all human sufferings was the "over-sexed womanhood tempting man as in the old Genesis story" (Steel 1929,290).

Colonial interactions between the memsahibs and the native women occurred through the multiple sieves of race, class, caste, religion and also region. The English women daily interacted usually with the low caste natives such as the dhobi, the mali, the wet-nurse and the ayah. The upper class native women observed *purdah* and asserted on their superiority and sanctity during their interactions with their European counterparts. Women missionaries, who visited the secluded native women, wrote detailed accounts about their encounters. In all these varied instances of interactions, the European woman acquired diverse positions such as that of the missionary proselytisers, sexual competitors, domestic employers and also educationists. The relationship between the European women and the natives was not simply one of the powerful white women exercising control over the colonised females but more complex and contradictory. As her autobiography emphasises, Steel came in close contact with the native women while carrying out her self-appointed duties of giving medical advices to them. Amongst other reformative approaches, she vehemently tried to protest against female infanticide, which was trending in Panjab then. She was always energetic and took special interests in educating the women of her region. She started her own reading classes and finally managed to set up a school for the girls at Kasur. For a lady of her social position, involvement in the education of Indian women were unusual. This "civilizing mission" was supposedly the amalgamation of both the imperialist and the Victorian feminist agendas. In *The Garden of Fidelity* she states, "All my life I have been keen not so much on the rights as the wrongs of women" (Steel 1929, 265). At one point, she totally obliterates the plight of the poor white women and even the barrack wives under the banner of social reforms which she meted out to the natives. Though her actions can be said to be similar to those of other Christian missionaries, Steel was apprehensive about the latter's methods being overtly liberal. Her views on gendered attributes were often complicated and sometimes contradictory, the reason being her unveiled class biasness and also her tendency of prioritising British prestige in the colony. For her, the white woman was neither the victim not the hero in the mutiny but rather an intruder amidst the male arena of colonial insurgence. She blatantly dismissed the instances of sheer bravery shown by the only English woman present on Delhi's ridge during the conflict as "perfectly useless" (Steel 1909, 192). Steel was also totally unsympathetic towards the myth of tragic estrangements that the white women suffered during their stay in the colonies. She was highly critical about the European women's conduct with signs of impropriety or immodesty in front of the natives.

It is astonishing that Steel, being a woman herself, blamed her kind for cases of adultery, stating that "it is invariably the woman who begins them" (Steel 1929, 122). She condemned every instance of sexual obsession borne by town-bred women with the tendency of acknowledging the peasants as pure and the town people, corrupt. Such typical perceptions made her epitomise the rural women of Panjab as morally ideal humans, free from the clutches of sensuality. Steel observes,

> "...one must draw a sharp line of demarcation between the women of town and country. The peasant women of Panjab are on the whole, comparatively free from the obsession of sexuality. Not so the town-bred, whether Hindu or Mahomedan."(Steel 1929, 245)

Steel believed that the urban woman's preoccupation with sex was a characteristic device that defined Indian culture as a whole. However, she also noted that the Indian woman was modest than her European metropolitan counterpart and thus claimed "in sexual matters, despite the hoary old wickedness of Indian towns... the standard of national morality is far higher in India than in England" (Steel 1929, 247).

Like other European reformists, Steel voiced her objections against the social evils of child marriage, sati, polygamy and other exploitative practices on the native women. She also condemned the stunted lives of the Hindu widows but contradictorily, in the next instance, she glorified the Hindu practice of enforced celibacy on the widows, identifying the scenario with the lives of Nuns. In *The Garden of Fidelity*, Steel confesses her natural dislike for the 'sensual' in life (Steel 1929). She even regarded the *purdah* system to be selectively oppressive and emphasised on the notion that the *purdah* granted women considerable power over her men. However, it is important to observe that purdah had several implications on the lives of women, especially in terms of their health. The confined circumstances with occasional unhygienic conditions and lack of sunlight led to serious ailments such as Tuberculosis, Osteomalacia and most commonly depression. To add on to the problems, the *purdah* women refused to be treated by male doctors and preferred to suffer acutely rather than be examined by a man. Saleni Armstrong-Hopkins, an American medical missionary elaborates upon one such incident inside the "zenana" of Nawab Khurshed Jah of Hyderabad where male doctors employed by the Nawab himself faced great inconvenience during the examination of his sick wife. The patient was totally hidden from the view of the doctor and only her hand was revealed for examination that too covered by the palms of the female missionary. From the year 1870, trained female evangelicals came to India to attend to such purdah women but with proselytisation interests. But after 1885, Dufferin hospitals built under the patronage of Lady Dufferin, made western medical treatments easily available for the purdah women while also fulfilling their critical needs of female doctors and most importantly, seclusion.

On the contrary, Steel's observation on the *purdah* system had a lucid imperious outlook. Once, she had to visit a *purdah* "nawabin" for examination as organised by a missionary but she returned only to reassert her British superiority at a perceived insult which she received from her patient. Thus, she commented "I have always held that the Dufferin nurses and the lady doctors were a mistake. They perpetuated a vicious circle by bolstering up the purdah..." (Steel 1929).

Steel, in her works exhibited great efficiency in portraying native life with all its intricacies and thus deferred from the styles of other contemporary memsahib narratives. Many of her short stories focus solely on Indians with a total exclusion of white interference. It has been very commonly debated, that her native characters are more enduring, picturesque and also interesting than her Anglo-Indian ones.

Steel, in her novel *Voices in the Night*, creates the characteristic structure of the "exotic native female." She invariably stands out in showing how women, irrespective of their race, and their bodies get perturbed by the intrusion of an imperialistic social ideology. Accordingly, gender politics becomes just a device to sustain the imperial interest in the colonies. Since, sexuality was a consequence of social interactions and positional constructions, there existed complexities between the coloniser and the colonised. Steel, in her narrative, brings out the site for the Indian bazaar which was utterly infected and infested with diseases and immoral activities. The British officials vigorously condemned these areas and refrained from even going near such places. Here, Steel creates the character of Dilaram, as a representative of the strong, rebellious women of the "bazaar." The "nautch" girls of such bazaars excelled in classical music and dance and earned a lot of money by performing in private homes and even in public halls. Several English eyes identified the nautch system and nautch girls as the sign of Eastern decadence and sensuality. As a missionary, Mrs. Flunner condemned dancing on moral grounds. In contrast, Elizabeth Cooper, who was a 20th century metropolitan travel writer, stated dancing to be extremely modest and also pointed out that it was the nautch girls who enjoyed real freedom in India despite the stigma of the impure woman that was endowed upon them. The most positive opinion by far was given by Anna Harriette Leonowens who said that the dance was a miracle of art and indeed a beautiful spectacle owing to the rare beauty of the performers. The English men were usually warned against such improper women and their morbid womb that carried venereal diseases and thus posed a great threat for the next generation of imperial masters. Sobrai Begum exemplifies yet another dimension of the "exotic female" through her denial of the patriarchal domains. She constructs herself an image of a "public" woman quite against her upper class family protocols and performs a spectacular show. Grace Arbuthnot's Victorian principles do not allow her to experience such a jouissance as the Begum and even after being the assumed racially superior memsahib, she feels challenged by the native woman's exotic figure. The memsahibs like Grace, were only allowed to play the stereotypical role of a British official's wife living with the perpetual fear of their fragile bodies being susceptible to the diseases of the tropics. The memsahib's reproductive role was rigged with disease and deformity during her stay in the colonial states. Tropical anaemia, which was the effect of intense heat, along with Malaria aggravated the conditions. Uterine infections and deformity of the white woman's body came as an indirect result of unjustified imperialism.

In this traumatic situation, the white women sought aid from Victorian medical treatise and also guide books to fight against the repercussions of such ailments. Gradually, the preoccupation of the Victorian tropical medicines became not only the preservation and restoration of proper health of the colonisers but also the regulation of the bodies and the medical discourses of the natives. Thus, Steel, in *Voices in the Night*, successfully brings out the caricature beneath the reformative agendas of the English coloniser.

Though Steel became thoroughly involved with the suffragette movement in the later part of her life, she had played a significant role as a colonising reformist in the Indian subcontinent. She cleverly balances benevolent imperialism with household management and further exemplifies the tactics for her fellow memsahibs. The question that needs deliverance is why are Steel's views on women rampant with contradictions? She never directly answers this but her works substantiate that she felt, favours as well as hindrances were inseparable modes of existence, disbursed to the fair sex in the colonial era.

References

Powell, Violet. 1981. *Flora Annie Steel: Novelist of India*. London: Heinemann.

Sen, Indrani. 2008. *Memsahibs' Writings*. Delhi: Orient Longman.

Steel, Flora Annie. 1929. *The Garden of Fidelity*. London: Macmillan.

Steel, Flora Annie. 1909. *India Through the Ages*. London: George Routledge and Co.

Steel, Flora Annie. 1896. *On the Face of Waters*. New York: Macmillan.

Steel, Flora Annie. 1893. *Miss Stuart's Legacy*. London: Macmillan.

In: Imperial Maladies
Editors: D. Bandyopadhyay et al.
ISBN: 978-1-53611-863-6

Chapter 13

THE CAGED PHOENIX? POLITICS OF AFFECTION AND IDENTITY FOR WOMEN MEDICS IN COLONIAL BENGAL

Sanchayita Paul Chakraborty[1,*] and Dhritiman Chakraborty[2]
[1]Department of English, University of North Bengal, Siliguri, West Bengal, India
[2]Department of English, Raigunj Surendranath Mahavidyalaya, University of Gour Banga, Malda, West Bengal, India

This chapter will attempt to shed light on the condition of women subjects as practitioners of medicine in the late colonial period in India within the structured and yet subversive spaces based on the intersectional registers of gender and nationalist identity. Science in general, and medicinal science in particular, was projected as the major instrument of modernity that in its colonial form entered India for the purported objective of civilising the mass, thus providing the most needed legitimacy in the

* Corresponding Author's Address: Women's College Road, Pirojpur, Malda, West Bengal, India. PIN: 732101 Email: sanchayita.dhritiman@gmail.com.

imperial project (Mukherjee, 2013). This ideological side of the otherwise scientific intervention in human welfare makes this entire arena smack of tremendous hegemonic and counter hegemonic possibilities which then found its close ally in the fledgling nationalist movement that gradually gained momentum at almost the same time. However, this register of women's standpoint adds a different slant to this whole critique of western science and its trumpeted objective of human development in the colonial discourse. It entails a different space of both critique and assertion of women agency sometimes in contradiction to the nationalist movement, which was largely male dominated, and championed the cause of a virile and robust energy considered as a pre-requisite in the making of the incipient nation. Therefore, this chapter in prodding this space of 'otherness' that harbored the dynamic possibility of continuing both an external critique of the colonial power discourses and an internal questioning of the patriarchal dominance in deciding the nature of indigenous women subjectivity, will talk of a different notion of 'outside,' placed at the interface of diverse frontiers. It both shares the anti-colonial moments that transpired in the politics of nationalist bourgeoisie, just as it engages with the women question in opposition to what Partha Chatterjee calls as the 'resolution' of the women question in the nationalist discourse (Chatterjee 1999, 120). It therefore takes the whole paradigm of critique to a much more intense and reflexive level of curving out a space of women epistemology which neither makes an unqualified association with the nationalist call, nor it buys into the dominant perception of seeing scientific prowess as a constitutive part of the colonial/modernity apparatuses imported to India in its imperial mediation. It engenders a different modality of critique which to follow Bourdieu's formulation of *habitus* and *practice*, is much more reflexive and negotiates the objectivist/subjectivist divide within the complex and layered field of anti-colonialism, nationalist imaginaries vis a vis women agency as subjects of scientific competence.

The question of gender identity is central to this imaginary of the 'outside' as it both negates the predominance of the scientific knowledge claim in the colonial establishment and contested the manufactured notion of 'Indian Women' in the nationalist narratives. It is within this double-bind of critiquing the Western politico-epistemic approach and the resultant nationalist resurgence that tried to resolve the women question, according to Partha Chatterjee in the domain of domesticity and home, this chapter shall address how there could be a possibility of a different paradigm of epistemology, its possible resolution of the objectivist-subjectivist divide and the constituent forces of women agency that in this interlarding discourses of coloniality, nationalism and patriarchy emerged as a disruptive space. What further needs to be said is how this space has been foreclosed, superseded in the subsequent nationalist call for nation building and the associated exclusivist agenda that consolidated the patriarchal imaginary of woman as a subject of collective honor with certain irreducible duties. This same nationalist agenda then increasingly debated the women question in registers that gave more valences to ethical and moral considerations whereas completely shying away from any attribution to possible scientific and rationalist potentialities in forming women subjectivity. Woman as a medicinal practitioner hence is a misnomer in that narratives as it nullified the projection of Indian women as exemplars of moral uprightness, thus reinforcing the epitomes of purity and virginity in contrast to their western counterpart. It is in this postcolonial invocation of Indian women as mother and sister with unparalleled aptitude and unmatchable integrity, the question of Indian women as capable of furnishing any scientific vigor was procedurally lost. The nationalist question thus foreclosed a whole space of scientific thinking that a number of women in their personal capacity participated and built up in distinction from their male counterparts.

WOMEN OUTSIDE HOME: THE ADVENT OF WOMEN MEDICS

Women's entry into the professional urban spaces first began with women teachers and women medics. It was necessary to incorporate more women into the teaching and medical professions to bring more women in the public discourse. The socio-cultural prejudice against women's public presence had been the major motivation behind the custom of *purdah* or veiling which reified a specific *habitus* about woman subjectivity within the spatial limits of home and family. The archetypal division of spaces in terms of gendered categories whereby women resided in the home, *antahpur* and their male counterparts were associated with the outside world was pervasive back then. *Veil* or *Purdah* hence turned into symbols of honor that women were expected to wear while venturing out in the public spaces. This socio-cultural norm was the main obstacle in the propagation of women's education as it was required of them to go outside to avail the professional school and college education. The British reformers along with the Bengali men who newly converted to evangelical sects within Hinduism like *Brahmos* vigorously promoted women's education for liberal emancipatory purposes. Predominant social norms also did not permit the co-education system and the professional, economic and educational equality between man and woman. Woman's education was envisaged primarily as the system of creating companionate wives for the new western educated urban elite men. Educated women were not expected to earn their livings on a par with men, sharing the same professional space. The construction of 'new womanhood' in this procedure maintained a perfect division between the 'home,' the *andarmahal* and the 'world,' the *bahir* and the world of the woman was strictly fixed within the space of the home. Partha Chatterjee formulates the division as the part of the nationalist resolution on the woman question in this way-

> The new woman defined in this way was subjected to a new patriarchy. In fact, the social order connecting the home and the world in which nationalists placed the new woman was contrasted not only with that of modern western society; it was explicitly distinguished from the patriarchy of the indigenous tradition, the same tradition that had been put on the dock by the colonial interrogators. Sure, enough, nationalism adopted several elements from tradition as marks of its native cultural identity, but this was now a "classicized" tradition-reformed,

reconstructed, fortified against charges of barbarism and irrationality (Chatterjee 1999, 127).

This conceptualisation of the 'new woman' did not envisage women in pursuit of scientific knowledge and professional degree.

Notwithstanding the emergence of the politics of negotiation and conflict that brought women outside the home, social prejudice against free mingling of men and women persisted. On the other hand, the subsequent higher education of women in schools and colleges made them conscious of the social and economic rights and ignited their aspiration for public roles. Women teachers and medics are the outcome of this long journey of women from the home to the world. Although the girls' schools and colleges gave a comparatively respectable space for women teachers, the struggle got tougher for the women medics as they were few to intervene in the henceforth male space of medicinal discourse, compared to their teaching counterparts.

Therefore, the relationship between gender and colonial medicinal discourse had been problematic for the inherent hierarchised binarism. The social prejudice against women's interest in science hindered the growth of women's science education. Women's inclusion into the medicinal science education was initiated as a part of the colonial and reformist policy of women's education and it is generated by the necessity to appoint native women medics as associates of the European missionary women medics in the medical institutions, hospitals and dispensaries.

The letter of Nilkamal Mitra to Bengal Secretary concerning women's inclusion in medicinal curriculum on 19th January, 1875 was an important document in this regard as he wanted to know the opinion of Lieutenant Governor on including Hindu women in professional medicinal discourse and discussed many provisions which could help in incorporating interested female students in medical higher education. The colonial Bengal was not ready until 1875 to accept women medics as part of the western model of professional medical education as the various documents showed the reverse opinions of Western male medics against allowing the native women medics into the professional medicinal spaces. The British government took the initiative to admit women in the professional higher medical education as they understood the necessity of women medics in introducing western medical care into the *antohpur*, the domestic Bengali world which would not allow the intervention of the male medics into the women's world due to social prejudice. 'Chikitsa Bigyane Mahila' ('Women in Medical Science'), the chapter in Binoybhusan Ray's book, *Chikitsa Bigyaner Itihas: Unish Satake Banglay Paschatya Sikhsar provab (The History of Medicinal Science: The Influence of Western Education on Nineteenth Century Bengal)* probed in detail into the growth of women's medical education in Colonial Bengal. But the official dictum was not enough to eradicate the patriarchal hierarchical subjugation which constantly denied sufficient space to the women medics, for her higher education as well as for her professional practice. Therefore what is evident from these separate works is how *antohpur* turned into a zone of conflict and debate that subsequently enabled the colonial discourse to facilitate women education in the medical discipline. This then transformed the existent *habitus* which was dominated by the patriarchal prejudices and paved for the emergence of a new identity of women medics.

WOMEN MEDICS AND THE POLITICS OF AFFECTION IN *ANDARMAHAL*

Medical treatment in a family and in a particular community is regulated by its own "cultural guidelines" (Kakar 1977, 7) which are closely entangled with the religious, social and political norms prevailing in that community. It also controls the system of medical treatment; the persons associated with this treatment and the family members whose authority supervises the whole procedure. When we look into the medicinal discourse in the colonial period, these "cultural guidelines" of the native community and its negotiations with the colonial scientific medicinal discourse offers a significant interface, within which the question of woman medic is situated. The woman question is one of the important sites to reify colonial civilising mission, emboldened by the narrative of the 'degenerated' situation of the native woman. It is important to note that though the colonial critique of the Hindu and Muslim women's condition did negotiate with the socio-religious issues like child-marriage, the custom of Sati, widow-remarriage and *koulinya* custom but it did not intervene in the health issues of the Hindu and Muslim women. In fact, the British colonial power was not interested in the health concerns of the colonised woman because of its entanglements with the politics of domesticity and seclusion resulting in the strategic apathy to intrude into the *andarmahal*, the private space of the women, which was considered to be the separated *zenana* even for the native men. The Christian missionary women were the first witness to the native woman's health concerns as they were introduced to the Indian domestic world as the teacher. Their observations and reports to the Viceroy's and Governor's wives were the first communicating sites between the colonial medicinal discourse and the traditional medical system. These documents provided another point of justification for the colonial civilizing mission and, simultaneously it also necessitated a hegemonic control of the British over the ancient medicinal discourse of India. Thus, a dual hierarchy is established through the supremacy of the British medicinal discourse over the traditional Indian medicinal treatment and the proliferation of the Christian missionary imagination of woman's treatment which marginalized the elementary medical care of the traditional *Dhai* or the experienced woman associate during the birthing-process as 'grossly unscientific and unhygienic'. The *dhais* were not only the important helping hands during the child birth in the upper and middle class households alike, but they were also the primary caregivers, the only companion during the long process of purity and pollution customs part of the childbirth. Hence they asserted a certain agency composed of affection and attachment through their performance of traditional social norms and religious customs. Moreover, they had the only right to enter into the secluded space of the *andarmahal* of woman. In spite of their almost indispensable status in the birthing process, they were not entitled to the same valuation as the male medics. What is more significant is that the traditional medical discourses like Ayurveda and

Unanai also gave importance to the role of the *dhai*. The marginalisation of the *dhai* as the primary woman medic as she refused to realign herself with the western medical training of the midwifery was subsequently followed by the redefinition of the woman medic who was trained in the western medical 'scientific' and 'rational' discourse. This gradual emphasis on rationality did not take into account the salience of emotion and care-giving so significantly part of the traditional medical discourse. Therefore, the figure of the *dhai* held testimony to the limits of the project of training woman medic in the western model of impersonal and rational education. This represents a structure of subordination where the *dhai* became the subaltern gendered subject excluded in the colonial imaginary of a woman medic.

Actually, the institutionalisation of Western medicinal discourses in the early nineteenth century was facilitated by western missionaries, philanthropists, British imperialists as well as Indian reformers. The advent of the Western medical scientific knowledge was proliferated through the establishments of medical institutions and treatment. Western medical treatment was introduced in the colonial India as a part of the obligatory civilising mission which could not afford to be blind to the health concerns of the native Indian. The native medics, initially men, found their space in the western medical institutions as an associate of the European medical practitioners because it lowered the cost of the medical treatment. Western medical discourse found its major support among the western educated urban elite men who bought the discourse of the superior scientific Western medical care over the prevalent customs and medical care. The companionate wives of the urban upper and middle class men who were mostly educated by the Christian missionaries and in the newly situated schools and colleges introduced themselves as the 'new woman' and prioritized the western medical treatment over the traditional intervention of the *dhai*. The *dhai* had never been given the status of the woman medic, though she is the primary one to provide the basic medical care during the child-birth. On the other hand, it became apparent that though the native upper class women sought medical treatment in the western medical institutions, they were quite less in number in comparison to the native male patients treated in the western hospitals, dispensaries and institutions. This generated a necessity of the women medics so that medical treatment could be provided to the native women at large. Therefore, the new woman's alignment with the colonial medical discourse and its supportive documents in the woman's magazines and journals offered dual projections. On the one hand, it provided a sort of legitimacy to the western missionary woman's conceptualisations of the Indian women's *andarmahal* and thus created a space for the western medicinal intervention in the *andarmahal*. On the other hand, it also pioneered the Indian women's inclusion within the western medical discourse as professional women medics. Nevertheless, it underlines the supremacy of the colonial medicinal discourse over the traditional medical care provided by the *dhai* to the native women. Through this double-edged move of strategic compliance and contestations to the western medical discourse, we will attempt to understand the problematic interface between women medics and the western medical power structure.

WOMEN AND MEDICINE: INTERVENTIONS INTO A PATRIARCHAL SPACE

In spite of these multilayered oppositions, the mid-nineteenth century saw the rise of women students in the study of science and medicines. The Brahmo contribution was important to consider in this regard as they were the pioneering figures who not only initiated the science education for women in schools and colleges, but the first women medics also hailed from the Brahmo and the native converted Christians families. The incorporation of women as medics as well as target patients was the part of socialist reformation and civilising agenda as the British officials increasingly felt the need to incorporate women medics in the health-care system to provide medical support to women and children who remained outside the formal healthcare system due to socio-religious prejudice. Simultaneously it emboldened the colonial project of western cultural hegemonic homogenisation-the politics which marginalised the traditional roles of women as midwife and primary care-giver. The progressive Indian male reformers supported this project as it satisfied their anxiety over the intrusion of the male doctors in the privacy of the *zenana* as well as brought in the advanced medical treatments within the reach of the domesticity. This method of strategic inclusion and subsequent derecognisation of traditional medicinal discourses erected a hegemonic model of scientific medicinal discourses within which the women medics had to negotiate to curve her own niche, besides the normative supremacy and politics of authenticity of the male medics as well as the professional superiority of European and Eurasian female medics. The women medics, in their assertion of their professional identity, envisioned a new imaginary of the 'outside'-the space outside the nationalist model of woman's education and the subsequent 'nationalist resolution of the woman question' (Chatterjee 1999, 127). Simultaneously, they also voiced a critique of the western medical scientific discourse by including the politics of the emotion within their everyday practice as women medics in opposition to the inherent politics of rationality in the western medical discourse.

Hatu Vidyalankar: The First Bengali Woman Medic

Women medics were not the mere outcome of the colonial reformist policy of women's education and their empowerment through their inclusion in the professional arena. Women medics developed in Bengal in two ways. In one way, the normative presentation of femininity ascribed the role of nursing and mid-wife to women. But this was supposed to be inferior to the traditional medics like *Kabiraj* and *Baidya* in the ancient medicinal discourse. On the other way, women's higher education paved the path of women's participation in the professional medical training and thus gave birth to the category of professional women doctors. In this context, it became very tough for a woman to intervene in the world of traditional medicinal knowledge which was preserved for the male pupils. Rupamanjari was a woman medic at the end of the eighteenth century at the village of Kalaijhuti in Bardhaman district. Her father gave her the space to flourish her intelligence and scientific inquisitiveness to study the ancient medicinal shastras of Charak and Sushruta. Going against the grain, her father allowed her to be educated along with boys in the traditional *tol* or place of education under the supervision of the Gurus. She adorned herself in the male attire, might be intending to get incorporated within the patriarchal traditional medicinal discourse which did not recognize women's efficiency in the medical care. She remained unmarried and taught many students in traditional medicine. She was well-known as Hatu Bidyalankar. Brajakishor's acquaintance with this extrordinary woman medic during the treatment of his ailing mother motivated him in encouraging his daughter's medical education. Dr. Kadambini Ganguly, the daughter of Brajakishor bore the lineage of women medics by becoming the first professional doctor in British colonial Bengal.

The Pioneers: Women Medics and the Proliferation of Spaces

Women medical missionaries were the harbingers of the western medical treatment in the cloistered world of the Bengali *andarmahal*. British medical missionary's women provided both the healing of the body as well as the healing of the spirit, thus setting up the policy of 'double cure' for the *pardanashin* (Forbes 2005, 104). The first women medic in colonial India was Dr. (Miss) Clara Swain and Fanny Butler, who was trained in the London School of Medicine for Women, was the first trained English medical missionary in India. The notion that only the women medical missionary could intrude and provide medical care to *pardanashin* women motivated the medical training for women in Britain. It served the dual role; by offering jobs to the trained British women who were unemployed in their homeland, the feminist understanding of women's rights was transported from the coloniser to the colonised. It also reinforces the imperialist rule through the justification of the civilising mission.

Trained midwifes and women medics were in demand in the urban and district hospitals, factories and plantations. On the other hand, individual families, even the affluent household who could afford the Western treatment preferred the traditional medical care and the assistance of *dhai*. Often the Indian progressive men put the onus on the *pardanashin* women who allegedly rejected the Western treatment in favour of the traditional care of *dhai*. The first instance of the patriarchal and colonial subjugation in the medical education in Bengal was Abala Basu. She, even after passing the Entrance examination in 1881, was not allowed to pursue medical course in Calcutta Medical College and was compelled to follow her medical education with scholarship in Madras Medical College. Women medics resisted this act of negation as they realised the need of the knowledge of the modern medical technology to provide proper care for various gynecological diseases which remained untreated because of social prejudices. This urge for higher medical education contributed in the proliferation of spaces for women as it contributed in greater mobility for women in various cities-sometimes for higher medical education and sometimes for their professional practices. Dr. Kadambini Ganguly and Dr. Jamini Sen even went abroad for advanced knowledge of medical technologies. It was also part of their strategic inclusion as they knew well that intense professionalism and higher knowledge would give them space in the patriarchal world. Anandibai Joshi sailed from Calcutta to New York to study medicine in Women's medical College in Pennsylvania in the very year when Kadambini entered Calcutta medical College. In 1890, Miss Bidhumukhi Bose and Miss Virginia Merry Mitter became the first Indian lady graduates from Calcutta Medical College. Their intervention into the colonial city space through their entry in medical profession opened the city to more women who ventured to move beyond the conventional feminine performances.

DR. KADAMBINI GANGULY AND DR. JAMINI SEN: TWO WOMEN MEDICS IN THE PROFESSIONAL SPACE

The life and works of Dr. Kadambini Ganguly and Dr. Jamini Sen present us the interface between woman and medicinal discourses. Through the conflict between their femininity and their professional ambitions as doctors, they project the tensions between tradition and modernity. Rituals and inhibitions which clouded the traditional domesticated feminine existence were at times at loggerhead with their scientific education in gynecology. Kadambini was pioneering in treading into the untraded world of medical science as professional woman medic. She not only practiced professionally in colonial Calcutta, she also travelled outside Calcutta and Bengal to provide medical treatment to women of aristocratic families. Her appointment as the woman medic for the Queen of Nepal's royal family was one of the pillar of in her career. Her pursuit of higher medical education even after her marriage with Dwarakanath Ganguly was not only a strong statement of her undaunted intellectuality but it also highlighted the role of supportive husband and fathers who went against the conventionality to provide space for women's emancipation. Her free movement in the public space, her horse-riding in her daily journey to hospital attracted the ire of the social conformists and the patriarchal godfathers. But nothing could divert her from her intellectual ambitions. She fought against the social prejudices and raised social consciousness for proper medical care for women and child. She was also quite vocal against the deprivation to the Indian women medics:

> The Indian medical women will miss all the advantages of such professional duties by their exclusion from the medical charge of important hospitals or by being placed in an inferior position there, for in the inferior class of hospitals, few cases of importance will ever go for treatment, and in the large and important hospitals the major operations and other important duties will always be performed by the senior persons in charge (Forbes 2005, 112).

Her participation in the nationalist struggle, her speeches in favour of women's education and emancipation and her path-breaking efforts in propagation of women medics substantiated women medics' struggle for professional recognition.

Jamini Sen comes alive through the memoirs of her sister, the renowned writer, Kamini Ray and Dr. Hemlata Sarkar who was a classmate of Jamini. Like Kadambini, Jamini was quite conscious about the double marginalisation of the women medics-under the male medics as well as under the European and Eurasian female medics. She also suffered the economic discrimination in terms of payment. For the utter lack of independent medical practice, she was compelled to move to the Zenana Hospital of Solapur. After her two years' service in Solapur Hospital, Dr. Kadambini Ganguly helped her to get her professional recognition in Nepal's royal family as well as in the Katmandu Zenana Hospital. Jamini followed the path of her predecessor, Kadambini as she also realised the value of foreign medical degrees in finding recognition in her native country. Jamini's movement in Dublin, Edinburgh and Berlin and her professional medical degrees in these places reinforced her status as woman medic. At the same time, it also charted the struggle of a woman who left no stone unturned to get her recognition as a doctor in spite of personal depression, social and professional discrimination and patriarchal subjugation. What is more interesting about their struggle is how they negotiated their aspirations on intersectional registers of women as the subject of collective honor, the new epitome of nationalist pride and the often colonialist imaging of Indian women as backward, hapless victim of indigenous forms of patriarchal coercion. Therefore they collectively betray a different teleology of empowerment that can reflexively negotiates between diverse forces which are contradictory and mutually exclusive.

CONCLUSION

To get back to the issues raised at the very beginning of this chapter, this discussion has shown how a different modality of scientific discourse emerged at the turn of twentieth century toward women as medics and practitioners. The promotion of women medics both by the British colonialist reformers and the Indian progressives indirectly nurtured the imperialist civilising mission. David Arnold and Mark Harrison show how "Western medicine became a tool of empire: keeping white masters and colonial subjects healthy, facilitating social control, and creating knowledge that fed a discourse justifying imperialism." (Forbes 2005, 103) The women medics were subjected to dual suppression. On one hand they faced discrimination for being Indian women; the Western Medical discourse prioritised men before women, foreign credentials above native degrees, and did not recognise local languages and customs. On the other hand, their profession as medics opened them to the negative public opinions, so much so that they faced public caricature, derangement, threats of sexual harassment, rape and abduction. They earned professional prestige and economic stability on their own but it was not accepted in the traditional family and community values. They were the misnomers in the nationalist resolution of the woman question which resolved the public and private roles of women by celebrating their refined status within the home. The predominantly public roles of the women medics often compelled them to remain unmarried as the traditional expectations of Bengali marriage tended to become obstacles in the path of the women medics. This perception was emboldened when many pioneering women medics were forced to leave their medical practice after marriage. Abala Bose, Virginia Merry Mitter sacrificed their professional ambitions on the marital scaffold. This paper weaves these varied strings together to evoke some questions on the relationship between women and medicinal discourses and how women generate a shaping force in problematising the homogenizing patriarchal discourses of medical sciences. In this perspective, the paper relocates the works of women medics like Jamini Sen, Kadambini Ganguly as exemplars of how they both subvert the colonialist discourse on science and the nationalist codifications of women within the *andormahal*.

References

Arnold, David. 1989. *Imperial Medicine and Indigenous Societies*. Delhi: Oxford University Press as cited in Geraldine Forbes. 2005. *Women in Colonial India: Essays on Politics, Medicine, and Historiography.* New Delhi: Chronicle Books.

Arnold, David. 1993. *Colonizing the Bo*dy. Berkeley: University of California Press

Chatterjee, Partha. 1989. 'The Nationalist Resolution of the Women's Question' in Kumkum Sangari and Sudesh Vaid ed. Recasting Women: Essays in Colonial History. New Delhi: Kali for Women.

Chatterjee, Partha. 1999. 'The Nation and Its Women' and 'Women and the Nation' from *The Nation and Its Fragments: Colonial and Postcolonial Histories, The Partha Chatterjee Omnibus*. New Delhi: Oxford University Press.

Dan, Rekha. 2011. 'Chikitsa Bidyay Banganari' (Women in Medical Knowledge) in *Balaka: Sahitya Bishayak Patrika, Prak Swadhinata Parbe Nabachetanay Banganari* (Balaka: A Literature Magazine, Bengali Women in New Consciousness in Pre-independence Period) Issue, edited by Dhananjoy Ghosal. Year-20. Issue-30. Kolkata.

Deb, Chitra. 2014. *Antahpurer Atmakatha* (Autobiography from Inside Space). Kolkata: Ananda.

Dutta Ray, Mala. 2015. *Kadambini Gangopadhyay: Pratham Bangali Mahila Chikitsak* (Kadambini Ganguly: First Bengali Woman Medic). Kolkata: Signet Press.

Forbes, Geraldine. 2005. *Women in Colonial India: Essays on Politics, Medicine, and Historiography*. New Delhi: Chronicle Books.

Ganguly, Kadambini. March 7, 1891. "The Zenana Hospital and Suggestions to the Committee," The Bengalee as cited in Geraldine Forbes. 2005. *Women in Colonial India: Essays on Politics, Medicine, and Historiography*. New Delhi: Chronicle Books.

Harrison, Mark. 1994. *Public Health in British India*. Cambridge: Cambridge University Press as cited in Geraldine Forbes. 2005.

Women in Colonial India: Essays on Politics, Medicine, and Historiography. New Delhi: Chronicle Books.

Jenkins, Richard *edited Pierre Bourdieu*. 2015. Routledge: London and New York.

Kakar, Dwaraka Nath. 1977. *Folk and Modern Medicine (A North Indian Case Study)*. Delhi. New Asian Publishers.

Mukherjee, Upamanyu Pablo. 2013. *Natural Disaster and Victorian Empire: Famines, Fevers and the Literary Cultures of South Asia*. UK: Palgrave Macmillan.

Ray, Binoybhusan. 2005. '*Chikitsa Bigyane Mahila' (Women in Medical Science), in Chikitsa Bigyaner Itihas: Unish Satake Banglay Paschatya Sikhsar Provab* (History of Medical Science: Influence of Western Education in Nineteenth Century Bengal). Kolkata: Sahityolok.

Ray, Kamini. 2005. *Kamini Rayer Agranthito Gadyarachana* (Non-compiled Essays of Kamini Ray) compiled by Abhijit Sen and Anindita Bhaduri. Kolkata: Dey's Publishing and School of Women's Studies, Jadavpur University.

In: Imperial Maladies
Editors: D. Bandyopadhyay et al.
ISBN: 978-1-53611-863-6

Chapter 14

'LADY DOCTORS' IN COLONIAL BENGAL: WRITING, MEMORY, HISTORY

Pritha Kundu*
Deptartment of English, Chandrakona Vidyasagar Mahavidyalaya, Paschim Medinipur,West Bengal

INTRODUCTION

Medical education for women in colonial India started largely as a direct consequence of the missionary project undertaken by their 'European sisters'. During the late 1870s, the poor health situation of the Indian *zenana* or women became one of the major reformist concerns of an enlightened group of white missionaries who felt the need of engaging British women medics in the colonial service. At that time, the medical profession in Britain (and elsewhere) was under a male monopoly. The male doctors even kept gynaecological and obstetrical cases in their own hands, leaving only the nursing jobs available for women medics.

*Corresponding Author's Address: ChandrakonaVidyasagar Mahavidyalaya, Paschim Medinipur, West Bengal, India. PIN: 721201. Email: pritha_kundu2@rediffmail.com.

Dissatisfied with such gender-discrimination at home, some of these female doctors readily accepted the better opportunities to use their medical skill through missionary works in the colonies. Such missionary doctors assumed a significant role in the campaign for the introduction of medical education for women in India. In 1881 the Maharani of Panna sent a message to Queen Victoria, through Elizabeth Bielby (a missionary doctor) urging the Queen to do something to provide medical help for Indian women. Dr. Frances Hoggan maintained that the existing medical system in India had failed to reach out to the womenfolk (Hassan 2011, 61). Dr. Mary Scarlieb, who came to India with her barrister husband, was also deeply concerned with the health-problems of the Indian women. She convinced Queen Victoria to support her cause, which became a turning point in the introduction of medical education for native women. The Queen did not get involved directly in the project of training native women to become 'lady doctors', but her support helped Scarlieb to promote the idea fervently. Scarlieb records such incidents in her autobiography *Reminiscences* (1924) which remains to this day a valuable testament about the social and cultural tensions involved in the history of women medics in colonial India.

The project was, however, not an easy matter. During the colonial period, women in India received the facilities of medical training amidst a long-drawn and highly contested debate among the medical officers, government employees and philanthropist-reformists both in public and private domains. The powerful objections from Indian patriarchy and 'tradition' were to be weighed against the claim of 'modernity,' trying to advance the cause of women's right to health and education. This had been documented in a number of letters, newspapers and petitions preserved in the colonial archive. These accounts amply show how the cause was viewed and negotiated by British administrators, European missionaries and philanthropists, and also by Indian reformists who took a special interest in providing medical education and healthcare for and among Indian women. (Forbes 1994, 515-16; Mukherjee 2012, 1).

Between 1880 and 1890, the written documents on medical education were primarily concerned with the unhealthy and pathetic condition of the

Indian 'zenana,' and the need for training women medics for serving those poor, uncared for women. For instance, the travel-journals and letters (1880s) of Lady Dufferin, who took initiative in giving medical education to Indian women, can be cited as examples, showing how during her travels across India she encountered the suffering of the native women in matters of health and hygiene. In *Leonard's Illustrated Medical Journal*, Mrs. J.T. Gracey, a missionary, wrote:

> ....it is a fact that very little has been done to alleviate the condition of heathen women.It is estimated that thousands of women die annually throughout the East for want of proper medical attention...All European ladies who have been permitted to break through this seclusion and within the veil have borne the same testimony.They all sadly tell of suffering sisters, whose diseases will easily yield to careful and skilled medical treatment, but who are doomed by their seclusion to the unrelieved torture of living death. (Gracey 1882, 62)

Narrin Hassan's book *Diagnosing Empire* has quoted extensively from Lady Dufferin's letters and journals to establish her concern regarding women's health in India (Hassan 2011, 83-85). The Brahmo reformers writing on the need for female medics also focused on the social and conventional impossibility of male doctors treating certain 'female diseases.' In 1882, the letters of A.W. Croft, the DPI, to the Principal of the Calcutta Medical College were also supportive of the women's cause[1]. However, the causes were not welcomed by all. The *Indian Medical Gazette* attacked the notion that women were being trained as doctors, and claimed that they were rather fit for being nurses. It revealed the gender discrimination within the medical profession. The Dufferin Fund was founded in 1885 for providing medical training to the willing Indian women, setting up female hospitals, and financially supporting the project. Historians like Geraldine Forbes and Maneesha Lal have shown that this initiative got mixed responses from the contemporary newspapers and

[1]Letter from DPI to Principal, Medical College, Calcutta, proposing the admission of women, 5 May 1882, WBSA, General Education, March 1886, A 5-7, quoted in Samita Sen and Anirban Das,"A History of the Calcutta Medical College and Hospital, 1835-1936" in *Science and Modern India: An Institutional History, c.1784-1947* (2011), edited by Uma Dasgupta, New Delhi:, Pearson Longman ,pp.496-8.

reports: some reformist Indian men were eager to lend moral support, while the conservatives denounced it as a kind of intrusion by the colonial government into the sanctity of their home. (Forbes 1994, 516; Lal 1994, 29-66)

By the mid-1890s, Campbell Medical School encouraged women in greater numbers (more in comparison to the poor number of female students during the initial years) to enter the medical profession. Among the accounts available from this period (1895-1910) we hear the voice of journals that were sympathetic to women's education and other rights – chiefly *Bamabodhini Patrika* which regularly published small articles on the female students who passed out from the Calcutta Medical College and the Campbell School. The colonial archive is apparently 'full' with such accounts – the reports and letters by British officials, writings by European female medics, and the views of Indian men, both reformers and conservatives[2]. What is more difficult to find is the voice of Indian women themselves who became pioneers, through several struggles, in the study and practice of medicine. Some information is available about the early lady doctors like Dr. Kadambini Ganguly (1861-1923), Dr. Anandibai Joshi (1865-87), and Dr. Rukhmabai (1864-1951). However, they had not left their own memoirs. Some personal letters by Anandibai Joshi are available, and they mainly reveal her private concerns and emotions regarding her ambition – going to study medicine in a foreign land, and to come back to serve 'Mother India.' The letters also throw light on her wonderful personality which combined her humble and loving respect for her husband that is typical of a Hindu wife, along with an individualist assertion of her dreams and desires, unusual for a simple and modest-living Marathi Brahmin woman in 19th century India. Her voicing of her own dream of becoming a woman doctor seems to be free from conventionality that shaped the general male bias against women's education in the society she lived in, but nor did she directly engage in criticising the patriarchy.

[2]For details, see Maneesha Lal (1994). "The politics of gender and medicine in colonial India: the Countess of Dufferin's fund, 1885-1888". *Bulletin of the History of Medicine* 68: 29-66 and Geraldine Forbes (1994), "Medical careers and health care for Indian women: patterns of control", *Women's History Review*. 3.4: 515-530.

Much later a novel was published based on her life, titled *Anandi Gopal*, by S.J. Joshi.

In the period between the late 1890s and the early 1920s, writing memoirs and diaries were not too uncommon among educated Brahmo ladies, and also among advanced and extraordinary Bengali-Hindu women. Nevertheless, memoirs by medical women construct a limited archive, out of which we are going to read at length two memoirs, one by Dr. Haimabati Sen, retrieved by Geraldine Forbes, and translated by Tapan Roychowdhury, and the other, by Kamini Ray (the well-known female poet of early twentieth century Bengal) who published a short biography of her sister, Dr. Jamini Sen in *Bangalakshmi* (Bengali Year 1339, i.e., 1932 AD.) based on Jamini's own unpublished memoirs and diaries. As to fictional representation, female doctors appeared in a few texts in the colonial period, of which the remarkable one is *Saguna* by Krupabai Satthianadhan, published in 1895. This was the first autobiographical novel in English, by an Indian woman. In Bengali literature, such characters – however small in number– began to appear since the late 1890s. And most of these representations were 'domestic' in nature—that is, lady doctors were viewed within the limited structure of family or the household-system, primarily as nursing and caring figures rather than contributing to a larger social/cultural history of colonial medicine.

LADY DOCTORS IN BENGALI FICTION

The 'familiarisation' of the female doctor-figure related to her personal/emotional life can be seen as a complicated issue in 'Himani' (1899), a short story by Prabhatkumar Mukhopadhyay. The protagonist is a Bengali Christian, but her kindness and efficiency have gained her trust and popularity among the female patients of the local Hindu households as well. Himani faces a professional and emotional trial as she comes to treat Nabadurga, the ailing wife of her own former lover, Manibhusan. The man is unhappy in marriage, he cannot forget Himani, and stays in his workplace away from his wife. Himani herself comes to call Manibhusan from his sojourn, apprising him of Nabadurga's critical condition. She pragmatically requests him to show no sign of their former acquaintance. When it is required to transfuse blood into Nabadurga's body, Himani willingly acts as the blood-donator. She refuses to take assistance from any 'superior' sahib-daktar, but relying on the ability of a newly passed out local doctor, confirms her trust in and solidarity with her native colleagues. The native doctor executes the blood-transfusion with success, but Himani feels so weak that she has to remain in bed, with a bandaged vein. Soon she realises that she is about to die. Seeing Manibhusan's suffering and anxiety for herself, Himani decides to donate not only her blood to Nabadurga, but her 'soul' as well, so that Manibhusan can love his wife after Himani's death. The story ends in Himani's suicide by tearing the bandage and opening her vein, and Manibhusan's subsequent fall into a mental disorder. Nevertheless, he learns to love his wife by virtue of a mistaken identity: now he calls her wife 'Himani' (Mukhopadhyay 2013, 255).

Self-sacrifice and nobility of heart constitute both aspects of Himani's character – her role as an ideal, dutiful doctor who can risk her own life to save a patient's, and her nature as a virtuous loving woman who can choose her own death in the hope of clearing the tensions in the married life of the man she loves. Within a plot of middle-class familial or domestic love, duty and relationships, Himani's personal and professional lives are entangled in a complex interaction, rendering her position ambivalent as far as the family-discourse is concerned. Her marriage with Manibhusan is not possible because he is a Hindu, married man. With shattered hopes of marriage and family, she dedicates her life to the service of the ailing people. Her decision not to have a 'family' of her own comes from her frustrated love, but it also alludes to the general course of the struggling life of those women – and they were not many—who came to the medical profession.

In real life lady doctors were also looked upon as 'alien' and 'lowly' even by theirintended clientele – the *andarmahal*– women of conservative Hindu households. Lila Majumder in her autobiographical work *Pakdandi* (*The Uphill Road*) recounts an anecdote about Dr. Kadambini Ganguly that she had gathered through family connections. Dr. Ganguly once had an experience which reflected the social bias against lady doctors: she was given a house-call to attend a case of child delivery, and after the work was done, the women of the house treated her like a midwife, calling her 'dai,'and asking her to clean the place where she was served food (Majumdar 1986, 102). They could not believe that any respectable woman could have been a 'doctor.'

In *Mahila Daktar: Bhin Graher Basinda* (*Lady Doctor: Alien from Other Planets*) Chitra Deb points out that lady doctors in the 1890s hardly had a happy family-life: either they remained unmarried, or had to suffer and compromise under a social/familial situation dominated by patriarchy. In course of time, the social and familial prejudice against lady doctors was somewhat moderated: they gained some respect, yet they were looked upon as strict, 'manly' and exceptional figures – not naturally fit for family. Prabhatkumar Mukhopadhyay's portrayal of Himani as a lady doctor is also doomed to a frustrated and unfulfilled life. Here, the lovable image of a 'lady doctor' in fiction has been created successful by adding a romantic note to make her de-alienated or less 'unfamiliar'. Himani's character is both image-making and image-breaking: she leads a dedicated and austere life of sacrifice outside wedlock, she has extreme self-control, but at the same time she carries within her heart a deeply emotional nature, the painful memory of a lost love, and a familiar and dependable relationship with the *antahpur* (inner space)-inhabitants of Bengali-Hindu households.

In colonial Bengal the female medics had to face innumerable odds and obstacles, yet the characterisation of the lady doctor in literary imagination was rather positive, however stereotyped. Kaliprasanna Dasgupta's 1921 play titled *Lady Daktar* presents Gangadasi as a caring and kind doctor who promptly comes to the aid of a pregnant woman, when her health condition requires immediate medical care. At the end, it turns out that the lady doctor was the first wife of the said patient's husband. She had been kidnapped and thought to be dead, and neither her own family nor the in-laws kept searching for her any more. Rescued by a matronly lady doctor she was trained to become a professional medic, now able to earn her livelihood and live independently. In this text, too, the female medic is shown to be excluded from a natural and happy family life. When Parashuram (the pen-name of Rajshekhar Basu) –distinguished for his wit and humour – portrayed a lady doctor, Miss Bipula Mallick in his 1924 story 'Chikitsa Sankat' ('Crisis in Treatment'), he also depicted her 'success' in curing the male patient by taking care of him for life, that is, by marrying him. She leaves her practice, and the author comments with a humorous touch: "Now she treats no other patients, but her husband alone" (Parashuram 1978, 39. Translation mine). For a long time, it remained a kind of general consensus that an independent and successful medical practice for a female doctor is antagonistic to a happy married life.

WOMEN, MEMORY AND HISTORY: A GENDERED APPROACH

Fictional representations, however, cannot be considered as archival material to reconstruct a social history of female medics in colonial Bengal; for that, one needs to focus on memoirs and autobiographical works. In his article "Between Memory and History" Pierre Nora comments that 'modern memory… is archival,' only so far as it can manifest itself in "the materiality of the trace, the immediacy of the recording, the visibility of the images"(Nora 1989, 13). The specific context of reference, for Nora, involves the 'sites of memory' in nineteenth century France celebrating its historical architecture: catacombs, monuments and the like. However, Nora's general approach is to read history and memory as two opposing categories, although towards the end of the essay he admits,

> …memory has never known more than two forms of legitimacy: historical and literary. These have run parallel to each other but until now always separately. At present the boundary between the two is blurring;… History has become our replaceable imagination – hence the last stand of faltering fiction in the renaissance of the historical novel, the

> vogue for personalized documents, the literary revitalization of historical drama, the success of the oral historical tale (Nora 1989, 24).

For this chapter, this 'vogue for personalized documents' is the key phrase. Personalised documents – especially memoir and autobiography are literary genres which, placed in a historical context, can be read as an alternative history where a subjective and more intimate kind of memory gives a new and interesting dimension to the otherwise objective and factual method of traditional historiography. Interestingly, 'memory as history' has also acquired a gendered identity in a sense that historical memoirs written by women had for long been labeled as personal, affective and even 'amateurish' in comparison with the universal, impersonal quality of mainstream history, dominated by male historians. Things have changed in the light of modern feminist history studies. Historians like Bonnie Smith and Antoinette Burton have taken major steps in the field of feminist historiography. In her book *Dwelling in the Archive*: *Women Writing House, Home, and History in Late Colonial India* Burton discusses the memoirs of Janaki Majumdar, Cornelia Sorabji, and *Sunlight on a Broken Column,* a novel dealing with partition memory – by Atia Hossain. She shows how in these narratives, the spaces of the house and the 'zenana' became the archive of female experience in national, diasporic and partition history.

Majumdar, Sorabji, and Hossain lived through the late colonial history and the upheavals of a period prior to the independence of India – a period troubled with the intersections of tradition and modernity, nostalgia and a radical quest for identity. However, Burton goes beyond the specific theme and context of her primary texts, and suggests a broader conceptual framework regarding the limits and possibilities of feminist history, as she argues:

> Far from being simply 'personal,' subjectivity is produced and lived as history… And just as "storytelling is the making and remaking of the gendered self in social relations," so is history implicated in the production and reproduction of women's cultural imagination (Burton 2003, 28).

From a literary perspective it is interesting to explore how these memoirs, very close to literary genres like 'autobiography' or 'bildungsroman' are able to project a journey in history, in which the private spaces like family and home are constantly in negotiation with public spheres like medical college, hospital, wards and chambers. In the west, the proto-feminist quest for identity and self-assertion found expression through women's writing of memoir or autobiographical novels (or 'bildungsroman' written in a first-person narrative), flourishing as literary genres in the nineteenth century. Charlotte Brontë's *Jane Eyre* is still read as a celebrated example of early-feminist bildungsroman (novel of growth or self-education) in English literature. Our question is: how far is it possible to recognise a trend of 'feminist bildungsroman' in the context of colonial Bengal, especially in the autobiographical writings by lady doctors?

THE MEMOIRS OF DR. HAIMABATI SEN

The memoirs of Haimabati Sen (born as Ghosh, in 1866 in Khulna, East Bengal) were probably composed in the 1920s, but remained unknown for a long time. The manuscript (originally written in Bengali) has come to be translated into English and published in 2000 – i.e., almost seventy years after Haimabati's death in 1932. This chapter ventures to examine the memoir as a different kind of archival material, where personal memory creates a notion of how to read history – the gendered struggle for education and financial independence, especially in the context of women's medical profession in nineteenth century colonial India.

Geraldine Forbes' 'Introduction' to the memoirs of Haimabati Sen, and a paper by Indrani Sen titled "Resisting Patriarchy: Complexities and Conflicts in the Memoir of Haimabati Sen," have provided us with holistic discussions on the narrative. I am going to focus chiefly on Haimabati's medical education and career, although some of my observations may overlap with those made by Forbes and Sen. Haimabati's father was a liberal man who taught her at home. At her generous father's house, she used to enjoy a life of free movements; but an early and unfortunate marriage thwarted all her hopes and dreams. Very soon, the death of her debauched husband left her at the mercy of her scheming in-laws. She also lost her guardian-figures one by one – her parents on the one hand and mother-in-law on the other. Deprived of home and property, she moved to Benares.

In literary terms, this is the turning point in Haimabati's 'bildungsroman' (narrative of growth and development) as she undertakes her journey by literally going out on the road—in search of a better and independent life. Interestingly, the traditional binary between 'independence' which is related to an extrovert, public life and 'homespun life' which indicates submission and stagnation (a gendered division, much illustrated by Western Feminism) does not work in Haimabati's story – her quest for independence and identity is also a search for a home, for kinship and familial ties. During her sojourn in Benares she was able to earn a modest but respectable living by working as a teacher to girl-students. However, she was always eager to find opportunities for better education. Learning about the Brahmos' progressive work regarding female education in Calcutta, she set out for the city. Her journey in search of education was replete with trials and dangers (ranging from crude proposals made by an old man to a rich employer's attempt to seduce her), which she overcame one by one, by virtue of her strong will and presence of mind (and sometimes just by chance). In fact, the narrative of Haimabati's wandering alone across the country seems to resemble a tale of adventure or a picaresque novel. We are left to wonder whether it is justifiable to draw a line between fact and fiction, personal memoir and autobiographical novel. Eventually, Haimabati came in touch with some open-minded Brahmos in Calcutta. In 1890, these well-wishers got her remarried to Kunjabehari Sen, a poor but 'idealistic' Brahmo missionary. Here one must remember that widow-remarriage was a disturbing issue in the late nineteenth century. Though it had been legalised in 1856, in reality it was hardly welcome among upper caste Hindus, though some Brahmos, either to show their progressive nature, or out of genuine good sense, were interested in this. For Haimabati, this marriage was important because it gave her a 'home'—"This marriage became a powerful bond in my life and changed its course. I now thought of myself as a householder" (Sen 2000, 239). Haimabati's memoir also shows that the Brahmo patriarchy, though apparently more liberal than Hindu male domination, was not at all so wonderful and magnanimous as it seemed to be. Her husband's irresponsible and indifferent nature threw her into a life of instability and poverty. The need of a stable income to raise and support a family turned her to medical education. She thought: "Many girls had joined medical schools at that time and I decided I would do the same" (Sen 2000, 290).

Before going into Haimabati's medical education and career, a brief survey of her predecessors may be helpful[3]. Although Kadambini Ganguly was the first female student of the Calcutta Medical College (hereafter CMC) she was not awarded the MB (Bachelor of Medicine) degree, instead she was given license to practice as a less prestigious GBMC (Graduate of Bengal Medical College). The first two female MBs of the CMC were Bidhumukhi Basu and Virginia Mary Mitter. They passed in 1890. Virginia Mary's career was one of compromise and sacrifice. She left her profession to make her family happy. The name of Bindubasini Basu, Bidhumukhi's sister and also a student of CMC, had passed into oblivion, but Chitra Deb has discovered from archival records that she actually received her MB degree in 1891, and stayed in Calcutta till 1906, before moving to Dehradun (Deb 1994,107).

The number of female graduates from the CMC was small, and the reason behind this was not only the conservative society but also the fact that the entrance test for CMC required a BA degree. This was accessible mostly to educated Brahmo ladies and Indian Christians. Geraldine Forbes suggests that the Campbell Medical School's decision to admit female candidates since 1888, created a better opportunity for ordinary Bengali women (Forbes 2005, 114). Even married women who had a basic

[3]Here I have given merely a summary of the early medical education for women in Colonial Bengal, drawing ondetailed works already done on this area. See, for example: "Education to Earn: Training Women in the Medical Professions", and "Medicine for Women: 'Lady Doctors' in the Districts of Bengal" in Geraldine Forbes, *Women in Colonial India: Essays on Politics, Medicine, and Historiography* (New Delhi: Chronicle Books), 2005; reprinted, 2008, 114-17 and 121-33. See also Sujata Mukherjee, "Medical Education and Emergence of Women Medics in Colonial Bengal", *Occasional Paper*, August 2012, 1-32.

education in the vernacular and wanted to have some kind of professional career, could get admitted to the Campbell School. This was the historical context in which Haimabati could pursue her choice of a medical career. At that time, vernacular classes to be taken by Indian teachers, were shifted to the Campbell Medical School, whereas classes in English were conducted by European professors at Calcutta Medical College. At the Campbell Medical School, students were trained in some basic or elementary aspects of medicine and surgery. Graduates from this institution received the VLMS degree which was inferior to the more prestigious MB or MD degrees conferred on graduates of the Calcutta Medical College (Forbes 2005, 114-17). Although they had to face several disadvantages regarding status, salary and threats of sexual harassment, the lady doctors passed out from the Campbell School played a significant role in providing medical service to the remote and rural areas of Bengal (Forbes 2005, 117-18; Sen 2012, 59). They had, after all, a great advantage that they "had grown up in Bengal, they knew the language and usually the local dialect where they practised" (Forbes 2005, 136) and found it easy to enter the 'andarmahal' for home visits. Haimabati's memoir highlights these historical issues in an intimate way through her personal journey.

Haimabati got admission to the Campbell Medical School in 1891, already a mother. The number of female students was four, while there were twelve males in her class. At the end of the first year, in her own words, she "stood first in the examination and was awarded two scholarships for this" (Sen 2000, 298). Later, in the final examinations (1894), she topped the class and was awarded the gold medal. However, Haimabati's success infuriated her male colleagues, and the way they reacted was a vulgar and shameful instance of gender discrimination in an educational institution in Calcutta, at a time celebrated as the period of 'Bengal Renaissance.' The male students were on strike, protesting against a woman's being qualified for the gold medal. The newspapers, too, joined the uproar, supporting the boys' cause. The issue grew out of control and the Inspector General and the Lieutenant Governor had to intervene. Both 'peacemakers' were representatives of the colonial government; they negotiated with Haimabati and kept her 'satisfied' with silver medals instead of the gold one she actually deserved. This patronising and compromising attitude of the colonial masters make us doubt the real nature of their 'civilising mission,' as far as the question of gender was concerned.[4] Nevertheless, the authorities were 'kind' enough to grant Haimabati's compensatory request that she would be given a monthly scholarship of Rs 30 in exchange for the gold medal; so that she could attend lectures at the Calcutta Medical College. This incident would have never been known without Haimabati's personal memoir as 'archive.' Even the *Bamabodhini Patrika,* a supporter of female emancipation, made a brief and safe report—

> Smt. Hemabati Sen has this time passed from Kolikata Campbell Medical School with special credit. She has received five silver medals for securing high position, and she is also awarded with the silver medal, given by the governor-general. (*Bamabodhini Patrika* 354, July 1894, 235, translation mine)

After a few years' struggle for private practice in Calcutta, Haimabati Sen joined the newly established Hooghly Lady Dufferin Women's Hospital at Chinsurah as a lady doctor "on a pay of fifty rupees a month" (Sen 2000, 325). The job also gave her free living quarters above the hospital, and she had an opportunity to run a private medical practice alongside. Her role as a doctor is also marked by a negotiation of spaces: the hospital and the female ward became her resort, her home. She records how it started with her arrival:

> The hospital was not yet open. The medicines, utensils, bed clothes, … were all lying in bundles…. I got things arranged in my hospital and opened the outdoor ward. The hospital had fifty beds and four female patients [transferred from the general hospital]… One of them was Phulkumari—blind in both eyes. Babuni was another: both her knees were rigid from rheumatism… The third was Kalidasi, she was suffering from tertiary syphilis… The fourth patient had goiter. (Sen 2000, 327)

[4]Indrani Sen also raises a similar question. (Sen 2012, 59).

The way she remembers the details about her patients is almost like keeping records for a personal archive. She was conscious of her position as the sole in-charge of the zenana ward, with all its problems and concerns. However, Haimabati's manner and language betray more intimacy and a sense of tender responsibility than authority.

The memoirs also give us a clear pen-picture of Haimabati's works as a doctor. Generally, she used to pay home visit to those women patients who were kept in rigid seclusion. If a patient needed constant medical care-giving, she would not hesitate to accommodate her in her own family quarters. Gradually the 'home' and the 'hospital' began to converge in her own quarters. She brought her motherly heart to the treatment of her patients as well. Every morning several patients used to come to her quarters and wait downstairs, she would come down with hot water and food for the patients and helped them to wash up. It is remarkable to note how she introduced a sense of health and hygiene among the poor patients. She also recounts how the intrusions of the male doctor from the nearby Imambara hospital (this person had some evil intentions to harass her), became alarming for the female hospital's reputation, and she had to lodge a complaint against him to the European Civil Surgeon.

Besides the dangers of sexual harassment the lady doctors had to suffer, Haimabati's personal narrative as a record of 'memory as history' also exposes other corruptions in the medical profession. Her most remarkable record which can claim entry to a conventional archive, was this: a girl of eleven died in the hospital after marital rape by her husband. It was like the infamous case of Phulmani Dasi (1890) which triggered controversy over the minimum age of a girl-wife for the consummation of marriage, as discussed in Tanika Sarkar's 2001 book *Hindu Wife, Hindu Nation*. This incident recalled by Haimabati occurred after the passing of the Age of Consent Act of 1891, which said that it was a criminal offence for a husband to consummate his marriage with a child-wife until she was twelve years old. However, Haimabati was forced to remain silent, to prevent it being reported to the police. A false certificate, issued by the civil surgeon stated that the girl was fourteen, and the cause of her death was "septicaemia from normal menstruation" (Sen 2000, 334). For this, the civil surgeon received Rs 5,000; the assistant surgeon was paid Rs 1,000 and Haimabati was offered Rs 500. Morally outraged, she refused to accept the money, but her superiors bullied her to take it, despite her protests.

Haimabati's persona in the narrative reveals two contradictory aspects of her position and situation in the social and medical history for women in 19th century Bengal. In a sense she was radical – taking decisions for herself, rejecting Brahminical Hinduism, remarrying a Brahmo, and pursuing at great risk her ambition to get educated and become self-sufficient. As a lady doctor, she does not conceal her grudge against the monopoly and power enjoyed by her male colleagues. In one instance, the senior male doctor was paid Rs 1,000 for a case of delivery; and he gave the midwife Rs 100, while the lady doctor (Haimabati) got only Rs 50. Recalling this kind of gender-discrimination in her profession, Haimabati complained in her memoir: "Lady doctors and midwives were but pawns in the hands of the male doctors…when I thought of these things, I lamented the fact that we were born as women" (Sen 2000, 317). However, in her household matters, she played the role of a good wife and mother, who managed both *ghar* (the household) and *bahir* (the world outside) and continued to support her never-do-well husband, by handing over to him all her earnings.

The impression the reader gets about Mr. Sen is not a good one: initially he appears to be an idealistic missionary who married a widow considering it a part of his noble mission, but had no responsibility of a householder. Later in the narrative, the true colours of his male ego come out. He continued to abuse Haimabati for nothing and even torture her physically. At one point he got involved in a brawl with Haimabati's superior at her workplace, jeopardising her professional life. Haimabati had to save him from a legal action, by apologising for his conduct. He knew that he would never be able to earn himself, yet it was no longer bearable to his male ego to live on his wife's income. Haimabati does not use any harsh word to describe these feats of her husband, but her sense of irritation is not always hidden, though she tried to wear a stoical calm and accept everything as God's will. Her willing compromise with her husband's abuses shows how internalised the effects of patriarchy could be: being otherwise so self-sufficient Haimabati kept herself subservient to the man who, she believed, showed the 'generosity' of remarrying her and providing her with a respectable status in society. These contradictions and complexities in Haimabati's life, which Indrani Sen has also noticed (Sen 2012, 60), point towards an intriguing paradox in feminist history. Her struggle for identity, extraordinary despite all these contradictions, shaped her personality in two ways: by resisting patriarchy and by compromising with it.

MARRIAGE, FAMILY AND PROFESSION: SPHERES OF CHALLENGE FOR LADY DOCTORS

Regarding 'marriage' and 'family' – two factors that somehow affected or problematised lady doctors' career in 19th century Bengal – there are some general agreements that married women had to sacrifice their professional life to a greater extent than unmarried women. Virginia Mary Mittter's case corroborates that, and the sacrificial story of another married lady doctor named Sushila Devi was published in *Bamabodhini Patrika* (Deb 1994, 118-19). Dwarakanath Ganguly, an enlightened Brahmo activist who married Dr. Kadambini Ganguly, however, supported his wife's medical career. Kadambini had to confront more challenges in society rather than from inside the family.[5] Haimabati was a Hindu widow who converted to Brahmoism and got remarried. Although she had a long career, she suffered a lot. On the other hand, Bidhumukhi and Bindubasini Basu and Jamini Sen remained unmarried and were supposedly free to have independent and long careers. However, Jamini's life was exceptional which refuses to fall into so generalised a division. For Jamini, the notion of 'family' was wider, more nuanced and equally binding. She willingly devoted herself to a larger family which included not only her parents, siblings and their children but also a number of orphans and destitutes she

[5]The chapter by Sanchayita Paul Chakraborty and Dhritiman Chakraborty, in the present volume, discusses Dr. Kadambini Ganguly in details.

took care of. She had other kinds of problems in her career, in professional and gendered terms; and it was mentally very stressful for her to bear the agonies alone, due to her extremely introvert and brooding, sensitive nature. During her lifetime, her innermost pangs, desires and needs were hardly revealed even to her close relations, and she did not allow her personal documents like memoirs and diaries to be published. It was only after her death that her elder sister Kamini Ray published a short biography of hers, 'Daktar Kumari Jamini Sen' ('Doctor Miss Jamini Sen') in *Bangalaksmi* in the Bangla Sal 1339, from Baishakh (April-May) to Shravan (July-August). Kamini quoted at length from Jamini's notes and papers that were so far concealed. Her memoirs were written both in English and Bengali, and Kamini translated the portions which were originally in English, into Bengali. Although some of Jamini's Bengali writing were made available to us by her sister, her original English writings are difficult to come by. So I have no other option than to retranslate them here. The relevant issues of the periodical are at present available in parts at the Bangiya Sahitya Parishad Library, the Jatiya Siksha Parishad archive and the Gurusaday Datta Folk Art Society, in parts—which, when taken together, make a whole. In 2005, the whole text, retrieved from these sources, was included among Kamini Ray's prose works, published by the School of Women's Studies, Jadavpur University.

'DOCTOR MISS JAMINI SEN': A BIOGRAPHY BASED ON HER UNPUBLISHED MEMOIRS

Jamini was born in 1871, the second daughter of Chandicharan and Bamasundari Sen. Chandicharan was a Brahmo and supporter of female education, but he was against the medical career of women. He wished that his daughters would rather go for literature and teaching. This shows how even among the advanced Brahmos, studying medicine was considered less respectable than studying literature. The elder sister Kamini wanted to study medicine but stepped back with a sigh; she did not have the strength of mind to pursue her dream against her father's will. Jamini was different and more confident about choosing her own way. However, Kamini helped her sister in doing what she herself could not do, she supported Jamini to convince their father.

Jamini Sen entered the Calcutta Medical College in 1890/91 and bore herself in a manner that kept all discourteous male colleagues at bay. As Kamini Ray writes, "Her dignity was such as her male colleagues were hesitant of coming to her … even to discuss necessary matters" (Ray 2005, 62. Translation mine). Jamini passed in 1896 (Kamini gives the year as 1897) and tried to have a practice in Calcutta, but she found that people wouldnot call lady doctors in general; if only the male family physician was not available, a lady doctor recommended by him could be called. There was also injustice regarding fees. It was unbearable for the self-reliant Jamini to depend on male doctors to get a 'case.' So she went to Solapur, and then to the newly founded Women's Hospital in Nepal, in 1899. From this time, her life was also one of constant movement, trying to find a 'home' in the hospitals and among the patients she worked for, but never having peace of mind and satisfaction. In Nepal, alongside her hospital duties, she privately treated the Royal family. As a lady doctor, she had easy access to the *andarmahal* of Maharaja Chandra Samser Jong, and the royal ladies would try to get intimate with 'Daktarin Miss Sen,' but she would never disclose to others what she heard from inside.Kamini Ray as an educated Brahmo lady and a poet maintained decorum and propriety in her language, while describing Jamini's experience in the royal *andarmahal*. Under the colonial lens, the Oriental *zenana* was seen as a place of darkness, dirt, disease and scandals, which was 'notorious' especially in aristocratic and royal families. In this light, one may read Jamini's dignified silence and speech-control as a hidden archive, powerful in its impenetrability rather than its potential for disclosure. Due to her illness, she resigned from her job and came back to Calcutta in 1909.

Soon she felt the necessity of acquaintance with the new developments in medical science. Her patriotism was strong, and being an introvert and a reserved person, she did not feel comfortable at all to go to Europe and live among unknown people if it was not for acquiring better and higher education, and applying it to the health-care of the women of her country.As Kamini Ray quotes from Jamini's personal memoirs:

> Science is constantly developing but I have not been able to keep pace with time. The time so wasted must be restored. The scarcity of female doctors is a major problem in our country. Good female physicians are needed for gynaecological matters. Since my student life, Operative Surgery and Gynaecology have progressed a lot, so if I really wish to help my native sisters, I should learn the modern methods… study and observe them in specialised foreign institutions (Ray 2005, 64).

The clarity of her thought and the nobility of her motto are remarkably evident from her own writing. In 1911, she started for Europe. Her memoirs, unlike Haimabati's and like those of Janaki Majumdar and Sorabji, has some elements of transnational (if not diasporic) experience, at least on temporary basis. She agreed to write about her journey at her elder sister's request, but could not find time to write much. From Dublin she got the LM degree, and from Glasgow University passed the fellowship examination and was awarded the Fellowship of the Royal Faculty of Surgeons and Physicians. According to Kamini Ray, Jamini was the first Indian woman to be awarded this fellowship. The next year she went to Berlin to have further experience in the processes of treatment and surgery. The sudden death of her adopted daughter caused her to return from Berlin. This girl was a strong bond for an unmarried 'mother' like Jamini, and her death was a severe blow which almost shattered her, made her doubtful of God's Grace, and finally led her through a traumatic phase to a spiritual and philosophical understanding of life. To illustrate this, Kamini Ray quotes at length from Jamini's own memoir, which being too personal, may not reflect any historical concern or even facts about her medical career, but will provide an insight into her heart. Jamini wrote this portion of her memoir on her return sea-voyage. She was by that time exhausted of lamenting her loss, and God's injustice on her lonely life.The sea—the archetypal symbol of the ebb and tide of mortal life – had however a soothing effect on her soul. One night, she had a dream: a Divine Presence seemed to be consoling her –

> "Listen, my child," said that glorious divine personality, "no good work goes futile. ... You are given tenderness, affection and sympathy: dedicate these to the noblest cause ...
>
> The soul is immortal, she (the dead child) will live in your memory. For her sake, try to bring happiness to other children, so that she, though 'dead' for this world, will remain in your heart as an inspiration for your noble work (Ray 2005, 67).

This dream-experience inspired her to extend the idea of 'home' and 'family' into her professional responsibilities viewed in humanitarian ways. She took under her care many destitute children, whose mothers died in her hospital, and who were not claimed by any other guardian. She built a house named 'Vishramkutir' in Puri, where she provided a shelter to these children, herself bearing the expense of their education, and often staying with them on leave.

Coming back from Berlin, Jamini Sen joined the Womens' Medical Service (WMS) and in 1914, she was transferred to Agra. The whole tenure of her service is a story of displacement. She was transferred several times from one place to another, without proper reason or justice, only to serve the interest of the colonial authorities. This will reveal the helpless situation ofthe native lady doctors, though some of them, like Jamini were as much or even better qualified in relation to their British counterparts in India. Three British lady doctors, due to some misconduct on their part or unpleasant incidents, were transferred from Agra to Simla in summer, and Jamini was sent in their stead. Six months later, when Jamini got settled there, the 'problem' regarding the white ladies was solved, they came back to Agra and Jamini was transferred to Simla in that winter. In Simla, she found that no arrangements had been made for her living. She got two unused and locked rooms in the hospital cleaned and made worthy of habitation, and devoted herself to develop the infrastructure of the hospital. Her dedication to her work was such that she often considered the precincts of the hospital her temporary home. Wherever she was transferred, she was especially careful of creating a healthy architecture around her professional identity, building new blocks, indoor and outdoor wards, saving money for buying necessary furniture like operation tables – as if, the hospital-space was her own ‘home’. The detailed account of these matters in her memoir may be seen as a different kind of architectural construction of ‘archive’ in which she invested her sincerity and dedication.

Jamini Sen hated to be a sycophant to the white authorities, and this created problems for her. Despite her popularity and good work at the hospital, she was again transferred to Shikarpur in 1916. The period of her service in Shikarpur is significant because it is at this time that Jamini tried to make some regular entries in her personal ‘archive.’ She described in detail what improvements were made in the hospital in her time, which was later discovered by her sister in a file stowed away with a seal “Not to be opened” embossed on it. In those private documents, she recorded her work in order to judge herself, and make further decision concerning whether to stay there for the sake of her patients or ask for a transfer as the weather of Shikarpur did not suit her own health. This record, made available through her sister, speaks volumes for the dedicated service Jamini and her native colleagues rendered to the country, whose work for the most part remained unnoticed by the conventional colonial archive. From Kamini Ray’s account, we also come to know what Jamini wrote on February 6, 1917:

> The hospital has grown unexpectedly popular. Ladies from gentle families are coming to stay in paid cabins. In 1915, there were 213 indoor patients, in 1916 the number has been 478. The most remarkable improvement is about the maternity ward… here death of childbirth due to septic has been a major problem about women’s health. In a short time, I have been able to bring consciousness among them. I have served for them and gained their trust. If I stay on, I will be able to help them further. Moreover, there is problem everywhere because of the British authority’s interference. Shikarpur is safe and free in this regard (Ray 2005, 79).

Due to a conflict with the authorities over her familial duties, Jamini Sen resigned from the WMS and went to Europe for a second time in 1921. She received a diploma in Public Health from Cambridge and a certificate from the London School of Tropical Medicine. Upon her return in 1924, she accepted the charge of 'Buldeodas Maternity Home' founded by the Calcutta Corporation. She worked hard to make this institution really a 'home' for would-be mothers – a well-disciplined place of care, health and comfort. She trained some nurses efficiently, and wrote a manual called *Prasuti-tatva* (*Thesis on Maternity-care*). Overwork and stress affected her health; she took leave and went to Puri for a change, but even there she was invited to be associated with the local hospital. She tried to fulfil her responsibilities until she was too ill and brought back to Calcutta, where she passed away in 1932.

SIGNIFICANCE OF THE MEMOIRS IN FEMINIST HISTORY

The two memoirs discussed here can be called 'archival' in their thematic negotiation of spaces– between private sites recorded in memory and their constant correspondence with the public life of the two female doctors writing their own lives. Neither Haimabati Sen nor Jamini Sen consciously meant to write 'history': for Haimabati there might have been a slight hope for getting her memoir published, for Geraldine Forbes found among her notes and papers an ambiguous reference to somebody who was interested to publish her poems and short stories. Jamini had never wished to publish hers. However, the historical importance of both memoirs, as writings by female medics in colonial Bengal, is unmistakable. It should be remembered that the notions of Western feminism should be applied with caution to such narratives in a native context. The idea of selfhood and a rejection of 'submissiveness' which is traditionally seen as a 'feminine' virtue, is a major preoccupation of Western feminism. However, both Haimabati and Jamini, despite their self-respect and dignity, exhibit a tendency towards an ultimate submission to some divine power. For a Hindu or Brahmo woman in 19th century Bengal, there was little contradiction between education, a scientific mind, self-dependence and faith in the Almighty, which may not be so easy to reconcile for a modern feminist trained in the Western ideas.

In feminist terms, Haimabati's memoir is a story of rare courage, integrity and self-reliance of a 19th century woman from a rural and less privileged background than Jamini's. Due to her own sufferings and narrow escapes from sexual exploitation, she is sympathetic and open-minded to the problems of other women. Her opinions are quite articulate against the patriarchal oppressions in both private and public life, but her own compromises with the abuses of her second husband remains intriguing for a modern feminist reader. Regarding Jamini, only two points concerning the issue of 'feminism' are deliberately made: that she remarkably maintained her dignity and strong character during her student-life under the co-education system, and that she never tolerated the idea of being subservient to some male colleagues to get their patronizing recommendation for a case. Her struggles against patriarchy were rather subtle and intellectual. Probably because of her well-educated urban family-background and sophistication, she did not have to face the kind of crude problems which Haimabati had to. Her moves in career and decisions which are a testimony to her strong and self-dependent character should be read as symbolic stances against patriarchy – which may not necessarily be a male figure or institution but a symbol of authority and power. Her decision to study medicine against the will of a real father does not mean a collapse in the relationship between a father and a daughter, for Jamini remained otherwise devoted to her family, and her father seemed to have accepted her choice in due course. This choice is better to be understood as symbolic resistance. Likewise, her conflicts with the colonial authorities and the higher officers are important because the resistance came from a native woman of colour, who represents a subject seen as 'triply bound' by the structures of power in a colonial state.

CONCLUSION

Finally, it may not be wrong to say that the two memoirs speak with intimacy and sincerity about the conditions of medical education for women and works done by female medics in colonial Bengal from the late

19th century to the early decades of the 20th century. The nature of education and the kind of service for Haimabati were different from that of Jamini, but both tried, in their own ways, to extend health-service among the remote, the poor, and the secluded population of their native sisters. And for both lady doctors, the professional identity was ideologically or culturally enmeshed with gender identity – both of them, being married or unmarried, a real mother or an adoptive mother-figure, could identify themselves with the archetype of Bengali woman as nurturer and care-giver, enfolded in a 'home'-like space, within domesticity or in a professional workplace. The creation of a female protagonist's bildungsroman – though she is a lady doctor or a professional, seems to be inevitably circumscribed by the physical spaces of the 'home' in its different forms, within the historical and cultural space of colonial Bengal.

REFERENCES

Burton, Antoinette. 2003. *Dwelling in the Archive*: *Women Writing House, Home, and History in Late Colonial India*. New York: Oxford UP.

Dasgupta, Kaliprasanna. 1921. *Lady Daktar*. Kolkata: Emerald Printing Works.

Deb, Chitra. 1994. *Mahila Daktar: Bhin Graher Basinda* (*Lady Doctor: Alien from Other Planets*). Kolkata: Ananda Publishers.

Forbes, Geraldine. 1994. "Medical careers and health care for Indian women: patterns of control." *Women's History Review* 3.4: 515-530. Accessed August 24, 2013. http://dx.doi.org/10.1080/09612029400200067.

Forbes, Geraldine.2005. *Women in Colonial India: Essays on Politics, Medicine and Historiography* New Delhi: Chronicle Books.

Gracey, J. T. 1882. 'The First medical dispensary for women in Asia.'*Leonard's Illustrated Medical Journal* 3.3: 62-64.

Hassan, Narin. 2011. *Diagnosing Empire: Women, Medical Knowledge and Colonial Mobility*. Farnham: Ashgate. https://books.google.co.in/books?id=AzVnbcMMWwYC&pg=PA1&source=gbs_toc_r&cad=3#v=onepage&q&f=false.

Lal, Maneesha. 1994. "The politics of gender and medicine in colonial India: the Countess of Dufferin's fund, 1885-1888."*Bulletin of the History of Medicine* 68: 29-66.

Majumder, Lila. 1986. *Pakdandi (The Uphill Road)*. Kolkata: Ananda Publishers.

Mukherjee, Sujata. 2012. "Medical Education and Emergence of Women Medics in Colonial Bengal." *Occasional Paper* 37.1-32. Kolkata: Institute of Development Studies. Accessed August 24, 2013. http://idsk.edu.in/wp-content/uploads/2015/07/OP-37.pdf.

Mukhopadhyay, Prabhatkumar. (1899) 2013. 'Himani.' In *Prabhat Kumar Mukhopadhyayer Galpo samagra*, edited by Sudeb Mukhopadhyay, 247-255. Kolkata: Kamini Prakashalaya.

Nora, Pierre. 1989. "Between Memory and History: Les Lieux de memoire." Translated by Marc Roudebush. *Representations* 26: 7-25. Accessed July 7, 2010. http://www.jstor.org/stable/2928520.

Parashuram. (1924) 1978. 'Chikitsa Sankat' ('Crisis in Treatment'). In *Parashuram Granthavali, vol.1.* 24-39. Kolkata: M.C. Sarkar and Sons.

Ray, Kamini. 2005. "Daktar Kumari Jamini Sen: Sankhipto Jiban Charit" ("Doctor Miss JaminiSen: A Short Biography"). In *Kamini Rayer Agranthito Gadya Rachana* (*Non-compiled Prose Works by Kamini Ray*). 60-88. Kolkata: Dey's Publishing and School of Women's Studies, Jadavpur University.

Sarkar, Tanika. 2001. *Hindu Wife, Hindu Nation: Community, Religion and Cultural Nationalism*. New Delhi: Permanent Black.

Scarlieb, Mary. 1924. *Reminiscences*. London: Williams and Norgate.

Sen, Haimabati. 2000. *From Child Widow to Lady Doctor: Memoirs of Dr. Haimabati Sen*. Edited by Geraldine Forbes. Translated by Tapan Raychaudhuri. New Delhi: Roli Books.

Sen, Indrani. 2012. "Resisting Patriarchy: Complexities and Conflicts in the Memoir of Haimabati Sen." *Economic & Political Weekly*, 47.12: 55-66.

Sen, Samita, and Anirban Das. 2011. "A History of the Calcutta Medical College and Hospital, 1835-1936." In *Science and Modern India: An Institutional History, c. 1784-1947*, edited by Uma Dasgupta, 496-8. New Delhi: Pearson Longman.

CONTRIBUTORS

Debashis Bandyopadhyay

Dr. Debashis Bandyopadhyay is Professor of English at Vidyasagar University in West Bengal and was formerly a professor at Banaras Hindu University, UP. A Fulbright scholar, affiliated as Faculty Adjunct with California State University, Fresno, California, USA, he pursued research on the life and works of William Saroyan in the USA and as a Charles Wallace Fellow he worked in the University of Oxford, UK on the role of Goldwin Smith in the American Civil War. His research interests include theology and Psychoanalysis, Violence, Identity and the influence of eclectic Buddhism on the Western literati. Noted among his publications is the book titled *Search for an Identity in Ruskin Bond: A Postcolonial Review*, brought out by Anthem Press, from New York and London in 2011.

Anup Dhar

Anup Dhar is Professor of Human Studies in Ambedkar University, Delhi. He has a PhD in Philosophy from Jadavpur University, Kolkata. He current works involve a study of the interface of the Marxian political and

Lacanian psychoanalysis, and the question of 'transformative social praxis' in adivasi (and dalit) contexts. He is the editor of CUSP: journal of studies in culture, subjectivity, psyche. His publications include Dislocation and Resettlement in Development: From Third World to World of the Third (co-authored with Anjan Chakrabarti; Routledge, 2009) and The Indian Economy in Transition: Globalization, Capitalism and Development (with Anjan Chakrabarti and Byasdeb Dasgupta; Cambridge University Press, 2015). He has co-edited such books as Psychoanalysis in Indian Terroir: Emerging Themes in Culture, Family, and Childhood in India (forthcoming: Lexington Book's [Rowman & Littlefield Publishing Group] and Clinic, Culture, Critique: Psychoanalysis and the *Beyond* (forthcoming: Orient Blackswan).

Sambuddha Ghosh

Sambuddha Ghosh is Assistant Professor of English at Krishnanagar Govt. College, Nadia, West Bengal. He received both his Bachelors and Masters Degree from Jadavpur University respectively. In December 2014, he was awarded the M. Phil degree for his dissertation titled 'Between Other Fictions: Understanding Language Games in Jorge Luis Borges and Samuel Beckett'. He was also among the Project Fellows working for Project Bichitra, a website containing online Variorum editions of Rabindranath Tagore for the School of Cultural Texts and Records, Jadavpur University under Professor Emeritus Sukanta Chaudhuri, the website of which finally came out in June, 2013. He is at present working on his PhD dissertation where he is attempting a comparative reading of the poetics of exile in the poetry of Seamus Heaney, Derek Walcott, Joseph Brodsky and Nissim Ezekiel. His present areas of research interest include Modernism, the European Enlightenment, Structuralism and its Aftermath Postmodernism and Orality and the Epic Tradition.

Chaitali Maitra

Chaitali Maitra is a faculty member of the Department of English, St. Paul's Cathdral Mission College, Kolkata and a Guest Faculty at Presidency University (formerly college) and Bethune College. She has also taken post-graduate classes in the Department of English at Jadavpur University of which she is an alumnus. An eminent scholar in American literature, she has a special contribution to the field of American poetry. Her monograph, *Studies in American Poetry* (Kolkata: Books Way) was published in 2008. She has also distinguished herself as a book reviewer. Her reviews are regularly published in *Desh*, the celebrated literary journal in Bengali, and also in *Genesis*. She is associated with several social welfare activities, and takes interest in different kinds of literary and cultural programmes.

Abidita Goswami

Abidita Goswami is a Guest Lecturer in the Department of English, Budge Budge College, Kolkata. She also teaches as a guest faculty in Maheshtala College and Basanti Devi College. She completed her graduation from Asutosh College in 2013 and then received her Master's Degree in English from the University of Calcutta in 2015. Her research interests include Modern literature, Indian Literature in English with special focus on Partition Literature. Her research article *Colonialism after Decolonisation: The Fanon Perspective* (co-author Suchismita Neogi) was published in March, 2015 under the ISSN 2249-8737. Abidita has completed a dissertation paper on the fictions of Camus and Kafka, entitled *Meaningful versus Meaningless: The Struggle between Individual and Group Morality*, under the supervision of Parimal Bhattacharya over a period of six months in the session 2014-2015. Her paper *Education: Meaningful or Purposeful,* presented at an ICSSR Sponsored National Level Seminar, has been published in the book *Challenges in Indian Education in 21st Century* (ISBN: 81-89169-60-2).

Pabitra Kumar Rana

Pabitra Kumar Rana is Assistant Professor and Head, Department of English at Govt. General Degree College, Dantan-II, Paschim Medinipur. He completed his Masters from Vidyasagar University; and at present he is doing his doctoral research on the question of identity in the works of Amitav Ghosh. Some of his papers have been published in national level peer-reviewed journals. He has also presented papers in some national and international conferences.

Ujjwal Kumar Panda

Ujjwal Kumar Panda is Assistant Professor of English at Govt. General Degree College, Dantan-II, Paschim Medinipur. A research scholar of Vidyasagar University, he has submitted his doctoral thesis on the poetry of Dylan Thomas and Seamus Heaney. He has also published research papers in several peer-reviewed journals. His areas of interest include new literatures, modern and postmodern literature and popular culture.

Shreya Chakravorty

Shreya Chakravorty is Assistant Professor of English at Budge Budge College, Kolkata who is also pursuing her PhD at the Department of English, Jadavpur University. Her areas of interest include Victorian England, gender studies, subaltern studies and Postcolonialism. Her M.Phil. dissertation entitled 'Mahasweta Devi: Translated or Translocated? The Politics of Translation in the Renderings of Gayatri Chakravorty Spivak and Samik Bandyopadhyay' has been published twice, the second time being with late Mahasweta Devi's 'Bashai Tudu' by Thema, the publishing wing of Seagull Art and Media Resource Centre. The first publication by Avenel Press has been accepted by British Library, London.

She has contributed many scholarly articles in English and Bangla to renowned national and international journals including *Common Grounds* and *Alochonachakra*. She is also an active member of Bharat Soka Gakkai, the Indian wing of Soka Gakkai International - a global organisation for the promotion of peace, culture and education.

Suvankar Dey

Suvankar Dey is a Senior Research Fellow of the Department of History, Jadavpur University. Currently he is working on the history of Tuberculosis in Colonial and Post Colonial Bengal. He has worked as an assistant researcher in projects sanctioned by INSA (Indian National Science Academy), CWDS (Centre for Women's Development Studies). He is also a guest-faculty in the Department of History in K. K. Das College, Kolkata.

Prodosh Bhattacharya

Prodosh Bhattacharya, Professor and former Head, Department of English at Jadavpur University is an eminent scholar, with specialisation in Old and Middle English literature and language and Victorian fiction. He has formerly taught at Presidency College, of which he is an alumnus. He has a special interest in popular literature, genre fiction and cinematic adaptations of such literary texts. His PhD dissertation was on the novels of Marie Corelli. His papers and articles have been published in several academic and literary journals of repute. He is a very active and enthusiastic research-guide who is a constant source of inspiration to his research scholars.

Abhirup Mascharak

Abhirup Mascharak is currently pursuing his PhD in the Department of English of Jadavpur University, Kolkata. Apart from adaptation studies, which is his area of research, his other interests include Queer Studies, Translation Studies, Film Studies and Sports literature.

Piali Mondal

Piali Mondal has received her BA and MA degrees in English from Jadavpur University, and currently pursues a PhD at the same institution, her thesis tentatively titled "Violence as Dialogue in Early Germanic Literature". Her other interests are, in no particular order, Queer Studies, Children's Literature, and anything belonging to the genres of Horror and Mystery. She is about to join Jogamaya devi College as an Assistant Professor of English.

Suchismita Neogi

Suchismita Neogi joined Budge Budge College as a Guest Lecturer in the Department of English in 2015. She had completed her BA from Gokhale Memorial Girls' College in 2013 and then received her Master's degree in English from the University of Calcutta in 2015. Her research interests include Modern Literature, Subaltern and Diasporic Studies. Her research article "Colonialism after Decolonisation: The Fanon Perspective" (co-author: Abidita Goswami) was published in March, 2015 under the ISSN 2249-8737. Suchismita has completed a dissertation paper on Conrad's Fiction, entitled "Quest for Self: The Concept of Double in Conrad's Fiction" over a period of six months in the session 2014-2015. Her paper "To Be or Not to Be: Education Answers the Question", presented at an ICSSR Sponsored National Level Seminar, has been published in the book *Challenges in Indian Education in 21st Century*

(ISBN: 81-89169-60-2). In 2016, she also joined Mahestala College as a Lecturer.

Sanchayita Paul Chakraborty

Sanchayita Paul Chakraborty is a Research Scholar in the University of North Bengal, doing her PhD on interconnection between religion, caste and gender in Bengali Women's writing in the colonial period. She has contributed in journals like *Intersections: Gender and Sexuality in Asia and the Pacific* (Australian National University), *Global Media Journal* (University of Calcutta), *Cafe Dissensus*, and in books like *Different Americas: Resituating American Identity in the post 9/11 Third Worldian Classroom*, published by Authors Press, New Delhi, *Shaping the Discourse: Women's Writings in Bengali Periodicals 1865-1947*, published by Stree and School of Women Studies, Jadavpur University, *DE-CODING THE SILENCE! Reading John Stuart Mill's The Subjection of Women* published by AADI Publications, Jaipur, India and *Dynamics of Development and Discontent*, published by Bookwell, Delhi, India. She has presented papers in numerous International and National seminars and conferences.

Dhritiman Chakraborty

Dhritiman Chakraborty is Assistant Professor of English at Raigunj Surendranath Mahavidyalaya, (affiliated with the University of Gour Banga). Formerly an UGC teaching fellow, he is currently doing his doctoral research on *Postcolonial Political in India* from the Center for Studies in Social Sciences, Calcutta (CSSSC), affiliated with Jadavpur University, India. He was jointly awarded a minor research project funded by University Grants Commission of India, to look into the possible re-appropriation/politicisation of a folk-form called *Gambhira* in North Bengal and Bangladesh. The project is completed and currently under review for publication. His research works are published in journals like *Economic and Political Weekly, The Journal of Politics, Asian Journal of Research in Humanities and Social Sciences, SubalternSpeak: An International Journal of Postcolonial Studies, Writers in Conversation by Flinders University, New Academia,* etc. His jointly edited volume on *Post 9/11 American Identity and the Third World Pedagogy* has come out in 2014 from *Authors Press, New Delhi*. He is also an editorial associate of *Kairos: A Journal of Critical Symposium*.

Pritha Kundu

Pritha Kundu is Assistant Professor of English at Chandrakona Vidyasagar Mahavidyalaya, Paschim Medinipur. An alumnus of Presidency College and Jadavpur University, she is now pursuing her doctoral research from Vidyasagar University. She has published some of her papers in national and international journals, and also contributed to critical anthologies. Her areas of interest include Literature, Medicine and Bioethics, 19th and 20th century literatures in English and Bengali, American literature, Women's Studies, translation and creative writing. She has recently published a Bengali translation of selected poems by Constantine P. Cavafy. She is also the assistant editor of a peer-reviewed journal (*Middle Flight*, ISSN: 2319-7684).

INDEX

G

H

I

J

K

L

M

N

O

P

Q

R

Y

Z